Praise for the work of Meir Schneider

"As an ophthalmologist, I always search for the best way to treat my patients. Based on the Bates Method, Meir Schneider's self-healing system has complemented my practice in those cases where our traditional medicine has its limitations. The best treatment is the one that is directed to the patient's needs, and the best medicine is the one that uses all knowledge and not only a part of it. Traditional science and complementary medicine are tools that should be used together, focusing on a more holistic health concept."

— Leonardo Verri Paulino, MD, ophthalmologist and anterior
  segment surgeon at ABC Medical School, Brazil

"Schneider's method is effective as a complementary physical therapy for the eyes."

— Emília Ritsuko Yasuoka Assad, MD, ophthalmologist
  and acupuncturist, São Paulo, Brazil

"Working with my patients has verified that many sight problems get better and heal by taking up the right habits. Meir Schneider presents us with a complete guide to doing so. He helps us to regain our trust in the power we have over our vision and our lives. As he says in the book, 'We all can take the time. We just have to decide that we are worth the time and that the process is worth our while.'"

— Amelia Salvador, MD, ophthalmologist, Alicante, Spain

"It is wonderful how each new book by Meir Schneider provokes us to incorporate more and more of the self-healing principles into our lives."

— Laercio Motoryn, MD, ophthalmologist and homeopath,
  São Paulo, Brazil

"The knowledge and application of the self-healing method was very important improving my practice as an ophthalmologist. The results attained by my patients and with my own vision are proof of the importance of the union of traditional medicine with complementary therapies. I thank Meir Schneider for being such a marvelous instrument for my personal and professional improvement."

— Ana Cecilia Gois Franco, MD, ophthalmologist and anterior segment surgeon and naturopath, São Paulo, Brazil

"I had the pleasure to meet Meir Schneider and use his method when I was finishing my apprenticeship to become a Bachelor of Optometry in 2005. His holistic approach toward visual dysfunctions changed me forever as a professional. His concepts remain present in my appointments, therapies, and lens prescriptions. Schneider's work invites us to naturally preserve our organism and to practice healthier visual habits in this very technological world."

— Fernando Nassif, optometrist with specialization in orthoptics and visual therapy, São Paulo, Brazil

"There are many kinds of patients, but those who get actively involved with their own healing process can surely go further. When I met Meir Schneider years ago, I started to apply some of his techniques to my work and was impressed by the results. We must imprint our will and optimism into everything we do, so we can go beyond it. Congratulations, Meir, for one more book that brings us simple yet useful lessons."

—Mauro Rabinovitch, MD, ophthalmologist, São Paulo, Brazil

Vision for Life

Ten Steps to Natural Eyesight Improvement

MEIR SCHNEIDER

North Atlantic Books
Berkeley, California

Published by
North Atlantic Books
P.O. Box 12327
Berkeley, California 94712

Cover photo @ istockphoto.com / cinoby
Cover design by Suzanne Albertson
Book design by Brad Greene
Eye charts and red drawings courtesy
of Flavio Kauffmann

Printed in the United States of America

Vision for Life: Ten Steps to Natural Eyesight Improvement is sponsored by the Society for the Study of Native Arts and Sciences, a nonprofit educational corporation whose goals are to develop an educational and cross-cultural perspective linking various scientific, social, and artistic fields; to nurture a holistic view of arts, sciences, humanities, and healing; and to publish and distribute literature on the relationship of mind, body, and nature.

North Atlantic Books' publications are available through most bookstores. For further information, visit our website at www.northatlanticbooks.com or call 800-733-3000.

MEDICAL DISCLAIMER: The following information is intended for general information purposes only. Individuals should always see their health care provider before administering any suggestions made in this book. Any application of the material set forth in the following pages is at the reader's discretion and is his or her sole responsibility.

Library of Congress Cataloging-in-Publication Data

Schneider, Meir, 1954
     Vision for life : ten steps to natural eyesight improvement / Meir Schneider.
          p. cm.
     Summary: "Presents ten simple steps to relieve eye strain, correct vision problems, and improve eye health; includes a full range of restorative vision exercises"—Provided by publisher.
     ISBN-13: 978-1-58394-494-3
     ISBN-10: 1-58394-494-X
  1. Vision disorders—Treatment. 2. Visual training. 3. Orthoptics. 4. Bates method of orthoptics. 5. Eye—Diseases—Treatment. 6. Blindness—Genetic aspects. I. Title.
  RE992.O7S27 2012
  617.7'5—dc23

2012011110

1 2 3 4 5 6 7 8 9 SHERIDAN 17 16 15 14 13 12
Printed on recycled paper

Contents

Chapter 6
Pathology Conditions . . . 127

Chapter **7**

The Blind Spots of Conventional Wisdom . . . 171

Foreword

Whoever has had the privilege to attend a lecture given by Meir Schneider knows that one does not passively listen to his work. The audience members are immediately treated as students and invited to perform exercises right there in the conference room. According to Meir, more important than talking about his method is experiencing it; theory is only valuable when implemented. We are beings with an incredible adaptive capacity, and so is his teaching: simple, direct, and transformative. It goes beyond the barrier of predefined concepts and comes with the assurance that we can walk away from the passiveness of our routine actions and into the freshness of new ones.

This book is a mirror of his way of teaching. The interactive and dynamic contents express the author's quality, moving us away from the apparent security of restrictive visual habits, to experience new possibilities. Since he considers that we all can improve our vision naturally, this book is not destined only for those who have diagnosed visual dysfunctions; this is for all of us. As Meir always says, routine is the ultimate degenerative disease.

I first met Meir Schneider in 1992, at a conference for six hundred people in São Paulo, Brazil. He made such an impression on the audience that it became the perfect time for the first training course in that country. I took part in it, although I had no previous experience in the health area. To be a health professional was not a prerequisite for Meir, however. He wanted to keep his teaching open to whoever was up to working on himself. This closer contact with the technique completely changed my way of relating to my body and my cognitive processes. Soon I started teaching others, thus complementing my learning experience. A few years later, already working as a fully trained therapist who specialized in visual education, I felt an urge to deepen my theoretical knowledge and went back to school to become an optometrist. This skill gave me better conditions under which to appreciate the grandeur of the method—Meir's great ability to bring complex theory into something that speaks to us. After all, theory tries to explain what we are. And Meir translates it with rare intelligence and generosity. There is no hidden material in his teaching; it is all there, at the reach of minds willing to experience themselves.

This book is much more than a guide to exercises; it is an invitation to transformation. Good reading.

M. Fernanda Leite Ribeiro, optometrist and self-healing instructor, São Paulo, Brazil

Preface

The world may soon be faced with an epidemic of vision disorders, as hundreds of millions of humans who have been subjected to constant contact with computer screens, fluorescent lights, and excessively lit cities gradually enter old age. Tragically, although they seem adequately equipped to predict such a catastrophe, the existing medical establishment is not at all prepared to address this epidemic correctly. From my personal experience, I believe medical doctors often tend to suffer from their own form of myopia, a shortsighted attitude toward holistic approaches to body repair and maintenance.

In this generation we understand the importance in any successful endeavor of budgeting for repair and maintenance. If we intend to maintain the value and the beauty of any product or system throughout its life span, and to extend that life span for as long as possible, steps must be taken along the way to maintain the usefulness of all vital systems and to correct any defects that develop along the way due to misuse, neglect, or accidental damage. Human beings need even more attention than machines in this respect; we need nurturing.

I am happy that people are beginning to wake up to this notion, and that a preventive, protective attitude has already begun working its way into the human psyche. Every day, more people pay closer attention to the food and beverages they consume, to the environment in which they live, and to establishing general healthy habits like physical exercise. But we still do not spend enough time addressing the health and well-being of our eyes. That is the purpose of *Vision for Life:* to help people maintain and repair their vision as a way to increase the length and quality of their lives. It seems ironic to me that the scientific establishment might be to blame for the sorry condition in which we are finding ourselves. The success that optometry and ophthalmology professions have had in recent decades is largely to blame for our culture's laissez-faire attitude toward the health of our eyes. This has happened by correcting vision problems through prescriptive lenses and surgical technology without offering any alternative.

People often take it for granted that if something goes wrong with their vision, medical science will come to their rescue. And while this may be true in many cases, I am a firm believer that it is always better to prevent a disease in the first place rather than to simply wait for the system to break down in hopes that science will offer a solution. First of all, preventative medicine is cheaper! Compare twenty minutes a day of aerobic exercise, such as running along the beach or bicycling through the park, to the cost of a $100,000 surgical procedure to correct clogged arteries. Even factoring in the price of an expensive, luxury gym membership and regular massages, the preventative approach is still far less expensive.

We must commit right now to creating a health regimen for our eyes because the whole body is affected by eyestrain. The human eye was made to hunt, to scan the horizon, to look at birds, to look into the distance. It was designed to be engaged in a variety of circumstances, looking at different things at different distances and in different light. If we stare only at a computer screen all day under the same lighting, we lose the variation as well as the acuity. We lose the passion for looking and seeing the diversity of life around us. What then does this do to our bodies and to our energy levels?

So many people report that they feel exhausted in the middle of the day, that they need stimulants to revive them. We must remember that whatever we do with the eyes affects the whole body.

The habits that you will develop if you follow the exercises in *Vision for Life* can be the lifeline you need. You will reinvent your passion for life while protecting the vision you have and correcting the degenerative condition from which you suffer. Best of all, as with any kind of personal exercise regimen, these habits will impact your life in ways that transcend the utilitarian benefits of disease prevention.

Like the poet said, "The eyes are the windows to the soul." By connecting with our vision, we connect with light and darkness, with nature, with our physical environment, and with each other in fundamental, simple, and beautiful ways. Going for a jog doesn't have to be just good physical exercise; it can also be a welcome relief for the mind. It is a way to reconnect with your neighborhood, to break out of your routine, and to expand your psychological comfort zone. And the same can be said of learning how to blink correctly, practicing the scrutiny of details, looking far into the distance, and nighttime walking.

Computers have certainly done much to advance the quality of life in our culture. Yet, every year, as hundreds of millions more people worldwide incorporate computers into their routines, they expose their precious eyes to constant, unnatural strain and poor lighting. By straining their central vision to stare blurry-eyed at the screen, people forget to utilize their peripheral vision. They forget to blink. They forget to breathe correctly. They scrunch their shoulders and tense their necks. They squint, trying to analyze digital data. And instead of using the natural human ability to scan for images, they simply sit and wait passively for the flood of constantly changing images to come to them. Remember: the mountain did not come to Muhammad; Muhammad had to go to the mountain.

It is our joy and responsibility to personally make the effort to connect with nature and with our own human potential. We each must make the commitment to claim our heritage and our birthright, which is health, happiness, and a long-lasting, balanced, productive life. And it all starts with our eyes!

Our senses connect us intimately with each other, with our environment, and with ourselves, perhaps none so much as our sense of vision. When a person loses his or her vision, there is no end to what he or she will pay for a doctor to correct the situation. Sadly, however, many procedures performed on people's eyes today, including Lasik surgery, do more harm than good.

Compounding the problem even further is that many people's eyesight ratings are misdiagnosed at the optometrist's office because of the stress and nervousness people feel while they are having their eyes tested for glasses. Often, people are understandably stressed, and strain their vision out of fear that it may have declined. Their visual capacity on an average, relaxed day differs greatly from that when they are fearful and stressed. But when have you ever heard of an optometrist confronting this reality? When has your optometrist massaged your shoulders and asked you to breathe deeply before measuring your eyes? When has your ophthalmologist asked you to pray or meditate (sing or dance) prior to measuring your eye pressure?

Most optometrists make no effort to test their patients' vision under normal, less stressful circumstances. And most people have no capacity to test their own vision when they are in a friendlier environment. Consequently, most people's eyeglass prescriptions are incorrectly based on stressed vision! The result is that the eyes, having no choice, learn to accommodate the incorrect prescription, adjusting gradually in the wrong direction toward worse, not better, vision. In fact, most optometrists don't even think stress relates to poor vision at all.

My personal experience in working with thousands of students and patients contradicts what these doctors think they know. Stress and poor vision do indeed go hand in hand.

So I advise my patients and students to sometimes take their lenses off while practicing the techniques I teach them, and I advise readers of this book to do the same. When you are in a safe environment, do the exercises in this book with your glasses off periodically.

It is no different from learning to walk again after a leg injury. If you never let go of the crutches, your legs can never regain their strength and improve to their full potential. Therefore, work out your eyes the same ways in which you work out the rest of your body at the gym, but remember to do it with great relaxation.

The exercises in this book are intended to help you to create a basic, fundamentally healthy routine that you can incorporate into your life immediately. If enough of us practice these exercises diligently and follow the advice in *Vision for Life,* we can avoid the coming epidemic of cataracts, macular degeneration, and other degenerative conditions of the eyes that scientists predict are speeding toward our culture like a freight train.

Ask yourself what is in the medical establishment's best interest. To restudy the eye field and allow new ideas to penetrate from outside of the establishment, or to continue learning new methods with the old way of thinking? Is it to help you to heal yourself with only a minimal investment of time and effort, or to tell you it is okay to have unhealthy habits, because they know how to fix you when you break? I am not trying to be accusatory or conspiratorial. I am simply attempting to rephrase the wisdom of an old adage that says you should never ask a barber if you need a haircut. Therefore, never ask an optometrist if it is possible for you to correct your own vision. The medical establishment is so dependent on technology and chemicals that it has little incentive to embrace a simpler, less expensive, personal, holistic approach to vision maintenance and repair.

This book is my response to this serious problem, and it is also my attempt to give human beings an alternative to becoming the playthings of profit-driven, surgery-obsessed mad scientists. You are your own patient first. Heal yourself using the techniques in this book and other books like it. Only as a last resort, or in the most serious of situations, should you seek the aid of chemicals and surgery.

For those of you who have perfect vision, or even better than perfect vision, now is the time to incorporate simple habits into your life to ensure that your extraordinary vision will be maintained for as much of your life as possible! It is my dream that all of us will have good vision for our whole lives.

List of Materials for Getting Started

Four pieces of dark construction paper cut 2 inches x 2 inches, 2 inches x 5 inches, 2 inches x 7 inches, and 2 inches x 9 inches

Masking tape

Tennis balls—at least two (preferably used—your local tennis club would most likely give you a few!)

Obstruction glasses (described in Step 8, pages 49–57)*

Red and green glasses*

Red pencil or pen (use a red felt tip pen if vision loss is extreme)

Plain white copy paper

Small flash light with red bulb or red tape over lens

Red and green playing cards (optional)*

Ten-foot and twenty-foot eye charts (charts included in this book)*

Flashing lights (when working with severe vision loss)*

Glow in the dark ball*

Beads on a string*

Pinhole glasses (optional)*

*These items can often be made at home from materials found locally, but you can also order them from the School for Self-Healing (www .self-healing.org). Email the School for Self-Healing at officemanager@ self-healing.org to order or if you have any questions.

Introduction

At one time, this book was to be entitled *From Blindness to Vision*, because I was born blind but, through years of effort and exploration, have taught myself to see. Today, because of this miracle, I can read, write, and drive a car.

The idea behind the original title was that my seemingly miraculous progression from blindness to sight would signal to readers that within this book are the resources anyone can use to improve their vision, regardless of their current situation.

In reality, I believe the great majority of this book's readers will not be those who are declared, as I was, legally blind. Rather, they will be people from all different points on the continuum of vision, including some with "perfect" vision who want to keep it or even build upon it. As dramatic as the first title sounded, I wanted to make certain that readers would not mistake this for a handbook only for the blind or severely impaired. So I gave up my attention-grabbing idea and looked for another title.

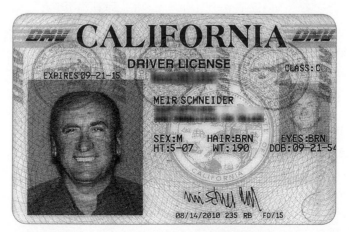

My unrestricted California driver's license.

Nonetheless, my personal experience in overcoming blindness remains at the core of this work. To anyone who doubts that improving his or her vision is possible, my story is a true testament to hope. Therefore, it was important to describe briefly just how this transformation happened. A detailed account of my life can be found in my earlier book, *Movement for Self-Healing*, which chronologically addresses the physical challenges I faced, as well as the long series of steps, discoveries, and exercises I underwent to overcome them.

Now I wish to summarize this same process with more emphasis on the psychological aspect. These emotional and spiritual challenges were central to the process of my learning to see.

The key obstacles that you, the reader, will face—whether you're legally blind or have the eagle eyes of an Air Force fighter pilot—will be similar to mine, even though the circumstances of our lives probably differ dramatically. The central challenge is for you to make a commitment to invest the necessary time to improve your vision and to expand your world.

It was difficult enough for me to do this in the 1970s in Israel, even with the burning, intrinsic motivation to rid myself of my blindness. For modern readers to make this kind of dedication of time in our hectic, hyper era, may seem impossible. Yet a commitment to doing it can pay off in two extraordinary ways: you will improve your vision while opening up your life.

Free yourself from the grip of a stressful routine. The amount of time and dedication I have devoted to improving my vision was extreme compared to what most people need, but that is exactly the point. Dedicate as much time as possible to these exercises, and remember that although your life may seem busy, making your vision a central priority is of the utmost importance.

Chapter 1

Healing Myself of Blindness

I was born in the Stalinist Soviet Union under difficult circumstances. My father was involved in an illegal business, taking and printing photographs for churches. This work could have resulted in his being sent to Siberia for twenty years. Furthermore, both my parents were deaf.

My grandparents on my father's side were opposed to another child coming into the family. At first, it was my paternal grandfather who had noticed that something was wrong with my eyes. After an examination by doctors, it was revealed that I had been born with cataracts. And although many people develop cataracts later in life, very few are born with them. I was, for all practical purposes, born blind.

In search of a better life for all of us, my family decided to flee the Soviet Union and to relocate to the new country of Israel. During this time of transition for my family, five surgeries were performed on my eyes. The first, done in Poland on our way to Western Europe, was unsuccessful. The other four surgeries—all performed in Israel—had scarred my lenses to the point that 99 percent of them was

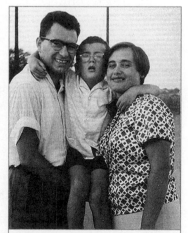

Figure 1.1. My father, Abraham, mother, Eda, and me, age five, looking and seeing next to nothing.

scar tissue, effectively preventing light from getting through. As a result, I was issued a blind certificate by the state of Israel, and most people in my life had resigned themselves to the idea that I would never be able to see.

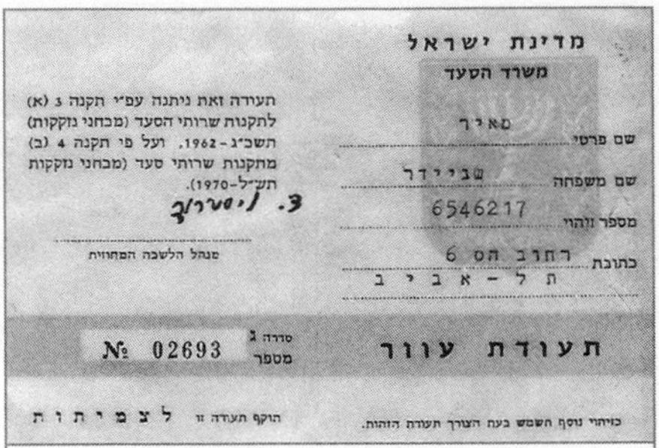
מדינת ישראל
משרד הסעד
שם פרטי מאיר
שם משפחה שביידר
מספר זהוי 6546217
כתובת רחוב הס 6
תל-אביב
תעודה זאת ניתנה עפ״י תקנה 3 (א) לתקנות שרותי הסעד (מבחני נזקקות) תשכ״ג-1962. ועל פי תקנה 4 (ב) מתקנות שרותי סעד (מבחני נזקקות תש״ל-1970).
מנהל הלשכה המחוזית
תעודת עוור
סדרה ג
מספר № 02693
כזיהוי נוסף השמש בעת הצורך תעודת הזהות.
תוקף תעודה זו לצמיתות

Figure 1.2. Blind certificate declaring me permanently blind by the state of Israel.

I was raised reading Braille, although I attended a standard school with normal-sighted children. I experienced much loneliness and isolation because of this situation. What do you do when you are blind, surrounded by normal-sighted people, and your parents communicate mostly with sign language that you cannot see?

My father, who was very interested in current events, often wanted me to listen to the radio and to explain to him what was happening around the world. He would have me listen to the news and repeat it to him, which confused me at first. I didn't understand why he had always lifted my head up when I tried to tell him what I had heard. I later realized it was because he had wanted to read my lips. But how would I know that reading lips was so important when I couldn't even see lips moving? This tragic comedy more or less captures the early days of my life. I was surrounded by confusion, frustration, and struggle. But I was also learning that there are many ways to overcome the challenges people face due to the circumstances of their lives.

It was obvious to me that my parents loved me. Still, our life was marked by fear and insecurity, having escaped the repressions of the Soviet Union, only to move to the young state of Israel, which was ravaged with war. Because of their deafness, my parents could not study Hebrew, which was so different from the Russian they had spoken before. Additionally, my maternal grandparents lost all the money they had brought with them from the Soviet Union on bad investments in Israel. Yet through it all, my grandmother steadfastly believed in me and was able to find ways to help me. She stayed with me in hospital beds after surgeries, when I was traumatized and feeling insecure from hearing many other kids crying.

Other members of my family believed that I should depend on social services. Although I didn't mind asking for money from my family, somehow I did not want to take it from the government. It was a deep instinct, the origin of which I understood later on as I matured. It is easy for a person who receives help from the government, as many with disabilities do, to develop a poor self-image as being needy or pitiful; it comes automatically, like it or not. But when you do not rely on that help, the image you have of yourself becomes stronger, and you are forced to become self-sufficient.

I was determined not to have the stigma of being a blind person. That basic resolve was the beginning of my transition and change, without which I would not have gotten to where I am today. As a response to the lack of security and uncertainty that filled my early life, I developed a sense of commitment. Kids often did not want to play with me. Girls would not dance with me at parties. I sometimes became lonely. But I understood the choice was with me to be depressed or to be happy.

So I escaped into my Braille books. With my books, I was in a different world and would read for hours on end. Even when my mother said, "Time to sleep, lights out," I would just hide the books under my bed. Although our walls were thin, as soon as

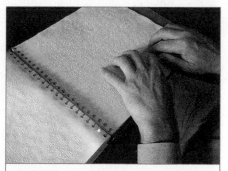

Figure 1.3. As of the seventh grade, I was the fastest Braille reader in Israel.

the lights were out and I knew that she couldn't see me anymore, I pulled out my books again and kept reading.

Whenever more of my Braille books arrived at the post office, I would hurry to pick them up. The books were huge. I was something to marvel at, a small kid carrying a very large school bag on my back, tied and strapped to my shoulders, with a Braille typewriter squeezed under one arm and a sack of Braille books under the other. More than once, the typewriter fell and broke, and we would need to pay to get it repaired. My father always resented the price, and I felt guilty about having let the typewriter fall.

Slowly but surely, my muscles built up. Many a passerby felt I was engaged in too much lifting and carrying. But that lifting, in many ways, formed my character. I imagined that, one day, something would liberate me from my blindness, and I acted by it.

I went from doctor to doctor, on my own.

I struggled against the resentment of the other children in school who thought I was receiving too much special treatment. They resented the fact that they had to explain to me what was on the blackboard. And I agreed with them! I wanted to be able to see the blackboard with my own eyes. I wanted to work on my own. I even had teachers that were mean to me because they felt I was not behaving right. They believed a blind kid was supposed to be submissive and passive—something I never was and, most likely, never would be.

I desperately wanted to be liberated from my condition. But all the doctors told me there was nothing I could do, that legal blindness was going to be my life, and that my vision would never be more than half of 1 percent without glasses, nor more than 4 or 5 percent with glasses. They said that I should accept the sight I had and that I should be happy with it. Those were nice words, but they did not work for me.

Discovering the Bates Method

My father was openly upset at the fact that his deafness prevented him from succeeding in life. My mother also felt like she was put down by the hearing world. I understood the prejudice they had experienced but, nonetheless, felt I had a bright future, though I did not know what it was.

Then one day I met another young boy named Jacob, who had dropped out of high school. He showed me eye exercises based on something called the Bates Method. I learned the eye exercises and started to work with them diligently.

To my amazement, as I practiced the Bates Method and experienced improvement, I received more complaints than ever from the authority figures in my life. You see, a part of my practice was to look from detail to detail; the purpose of this exercise was to stop my brain from being lazy. But my geography teacher would get upset as I moved my eyes from each bell beside the chalkboard to the other, looking at the details during class. She went all the way to the vice principal. Thankfully, the vice principal heard my case and told her that the exercises may help me, and that they did not disturb my ability to listen to her lessons.

My Bible studies teacher was upset that when my class sat in the yard reading biblical verses, I would close my eyes and face the sun, moving my head from side to side. When I faced the sun, my pupils would contract; when I moved my head to the side, my pupils would expand. My teacher said that it bothered him to see me moving my head from side to side, even though he recognized that I understood everything he was saying. He said that even though I was the best student in the class, I should stop doing the *sunning* because it bothered him.

Despite these reactions, I persisted. My retina started to wake up to light, and that was my vehicle to removing the thick, heavy, dark glasses that had made the world dimmer for me.

My mother was upset with the fact that I would run, ten times a day, up to the roof to do sunning. She said, "You are taking time out from your homework." Then she was upset that I would for sit three hours a day and do *palming*, an exercise to rest my eyes and stop them from moving involuntarily.

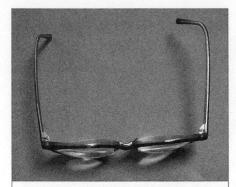

Figure 1.4. With these glasses I was able to read the largest letter on the eye chart from a distance of five feet (20/800).

In short, I encountered so much resistance to what I did that I didn't even know it was possible to attempt change without facing resistance. When everybody resists you, difficulty comes not only in doing the exercises, but also in dealing with the fact that your family, friends, teachers, and even neighbors oppose your efforts. Still, I persisted.

Within three months, I was able to see print. And not with 38 diopters, which is a microscopical lens, but with 20 diopters, which is simply a very thick lens. Headaches that had plagued me all my life disappeared within six months.

Seeing the Light

Within a year of practicing the Bates Method, I was able to see regular letters. I'll never forget the day I was doing the sunning exercise on a roof and looking at sharp black letters printed on white paper. I placed the paper at the tip of my nose. For the very first time in my life, at the age of seventeen and a half, I could see the printed word without magnification. This success took such a huge effort that I threw up. Again, I sunned and palmed and threw up, until I saw another letter, then another. Soon, I heard loud voices in argument. It was the neighbors downstairs accusing each other of creating a mess on the windows. I hadn't realized that each time I threw up, it was over their windows. So I went downstairs and told them what had happened. Instead of being angry with me, they were amazed at my honesty. I could have ignored my deeds, but I didn't. I was proud of the fact that I could finally see a letter. I honed my process and, within three months, could see multiple letters by putting the print right in front of my nose.

From then on, I continued to work. People were surprised that instead of just feeling my way down the road, I could literally see the road. Instead of not recognizing them, I started to know their faces. One neighbor was actually upset that I could recognize her! "What is wrong?" she would ask. "You're the blind person in the neighborhood. How can you see us? What have you done? What's going on?" It was amazing. I had taken away from her the feeling of security that resulted from her knowing what was going on in the neighborhood. It was almost as if she felt that the world she knew had been taken away from her. Here is the blind kid looking at everyone and actually seeing them. I was used to resistance but was pleasantly surprised by the first voices of admiration I received.

My diligence continued. I looked from detail to detail. People finally accepted that I could see and recognize them, so my status soon changed from being one who was nearly blind to one who was nearly sighted. I kept working despite the fact that my progress was slow.

A landmark came when Jacob, my friend and mentor on the path to vision improvement, told me I no longer had astigmatism. Don't ask me how he knew, but when I went to the ophthalmologist in the public clinic, she was shocked. She said to me, "I don't know how it happened, but you don't need the cylinders in your glasses to correct your astigmatism because you don't have astigmatism anymore!" I was not surprised to hear this.

It was at this time that I was taught the connection between the health of my eyes and that of the rest of my physical body. Another friend, Miriam, the librarian, taught me a series of exercises to improve my body. I began to practice movement techniques and learned that movement is life. Whenever circumstances block possibilities of improvement, there are always other possibilities that can help you to move forward. I learned from experience that the human body is capable of improving and healing itself. We forget that we have the potential to improve our vision. The world is so engaged in the myth that poor eyesight cannot improve, especially in a case like mine, that it is difficult to imagine a story like mine being true. I've proven the conventional wisdom wrong and have shown the power of healing exercises.

I am grateful that Miriam and Jacob taught me eye exercises and body movement and encouraged me to share these exercises with other people. I have met with people who have improved their body even from major conditions such as paralysis from polio, motor neuron disease, muscular dystrophy, spinal injuries, arthritis, strokes, and many other ailments.

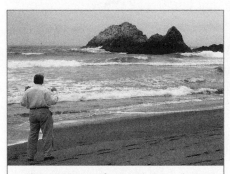

Figure 1.5. We forget that we have the potential to improve our vision.

I knew I had found my calling: to bring this consciousness to others. Most people have little faith in their own healing ability. My faith in their ability is great because of my faith in my own ability and my success.

There are two ways for me to describe how you can improve. One is to explain that the body has a greater functional potential than most people ever experience in life. The other is to demonstrate how to meet that potential through exercise. Whenever I work with people, I demonstrate to them that they can do more than they think. When they have pain, this means helping them not to let the pain restrict them too much. When they have tension, it means first helping them recognize the tension to its fullest extent, then decreasing it.

My own process was not smooth. My eyes used to move involuntarily three hundred times per minute until I learned palming: rubbing my hands, putting them around my eye orbits very gently, and

8

visualizing darkness. This would calm and relax my eyes. In one strange way, it actually helped me to have deaf parents in my teens. I could play loud rock and roll music, and relax with it. In spite of our thin walls, my parents couldn't hear it! Whenever I played this music, I would place my hands very gently around my eye orbits to relax my eyes. The movement of my eyes decreased to sixty movements per minute within three months. That's when my vision started to clear. The additional exercise of sunning warmed my eyes and started to activate my irregular pupils.

Although I could not exactly see, I gradually learned to look, even though it was sometimes painful. I had been taught by my Braille teacher to "feel the Braille and not look at the page. For God's sake, don't look, because if you look, you'll confuse your senses. You've got to *feel* and not *look*."

That order was so vigorous that I had learned to live a life without looking at anything. Looking was a new order to my brain. The result, even though I was starting to see more, was that my eyes hurt. Palming and lying down for a long time had helped me. Sometimes I just didn't want to see anything; it was just too much. But I kept looking.

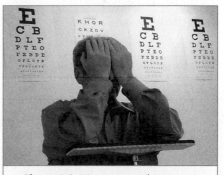

Figure 1.6. My eyes used to move involuntarily three hundred times per minute until I learned palming.

When I arrived in the United States, I met some people who were very interested in my work. They offered to help me train other people in my methods. It was new to me to have people embrace my experiences. I learned how to teach individuals—Miriam always taught me to work only with individuals—and how to teach classes in a way that would enable each individual to learn how to work with himself or herself. From this I learned that the greatest difficulty most people have is that they don't believe they can find the time to work on themselves. Most people think they are too busy. Others feel impatient and aren't willing to invest the effort it takes to quiet and to relax their minds and bodies. I teach them how to incorporate these exercises into their existing routines. I teach them that looking at details is something they had stopped being motivated to do a long time ago and that to do so stimulates the *macula*—the central part of the retina—and can prevent macular degeneration. I teach them that sitting with a loose neck is worth the investment of moving the head in a rotating motion before sitting in a chair. I teach people that while they use their computers, they should look far away from time to time to rest their eyes. These are simple habits that are easily incorporated into day-to-day life.

My own two children were born with cataracts, which was traumatic for me and for their mother, as we knew from experience the struggle they would face. At the age of two weeks, they went through cataract surgeries that allowed the visual brain to develop normally. This was not known in my generation. Because their surgeries were successful, they did not have to deal with the scarring that I dealt with when I was young. Using the techniques you will read about in this book, their vision has improved tremendously. Throughout their childhood and adolescence, my children have covered their strong eyes and looked with their weak eyes at objects in order to ease the strain of looking with the strong eyes all the time.

With an artist's mind and an artist's heart, my son is often in his own world in many ways. While in his world, however, he looks at details with great interest. Because of his powerful capacity of observation and love of detail, he sees much that others don't see. He has developed the best vision of any kid who was ever born with cataracts. He now sees at 20/40 without glasses. This is 80 percent of 20/20 vision, without his natural lenses. Anyone else without the natural lens of the eye would be seeing 20/400 (5 percent of normal vision). He sees 20/15 with glasses. Most other kids who were born with cataracts and had successful surgeries see 20/80 or 20/100 using much thicker lenses; 20/40 is unheard of for someone who has no natural lens of his own.

My daughter has also passed through many transitions. We used to play a lot of games in our living room, where she would cover her strong eye and play ball with me using her weaker eye. Seeing that ball as it rolled close and far made a huge difference for her, and her vision greatly improved. At the age of twelve, she developed elevated eye pressure. Immediately, the doctors wanted to give her eye drops to reduce her pressure. We declined the doctors' recommendation because we believed the drops could be damaging. I worked with her instead, and in spite of incredibly demanding middle school and high school schedules with many extracurricular activities, she found some time to work on her periphery, which reduced eye pressure. She also found some time to work on her neck. She saw acupuncturists and homeopathic specialists, took vitamin treatments, and got massage treatments to reduce the tension in her back and neck. I taught her how to relax her whole body in many different ways in order to bring more blood circulation to her head. Her pressure was reduced enormously.

The process was long, hard, and cumbersome, and had its ups and downs, but it worked. With high pressure, some people have a tendency toward developing glaucoma, and glaucoma expresses itself by damaging the optic nerve and diminishing the field of vision. So our success with her is partial but good; her vision is 20/20. Though her tendency is for high pressure, her optic nerve is very healthy, and her field of vision is excellent.

From these experiences with myself, with my children, and with thousands of patients and students with whom I have worked, I have come to truly believe that people can improve their vision and find the time to do so, whether they're in school or in the workplace.

A wonderful computer engineer, who once came to a class of mine, was able to improve his vision from 20/200 to 20/80 during the class. He reduced his prescription by half within eight months, from 7 diopters to 3.5 diopters. For the first time in his adult life, and still in his forties, he felt comfortable driving without glasses.

We all can take the time. We just have to decide that we are worth the time and that the process is worth our while. We need to make an effort to combine eye exercises with our everyday lives. Then we can thrive. Then we can excel. Imagine never needing to have any major treatments from the eye doctor. Imagine your life without cataracts, macular degeneration, glaucoma, or retinal detachment. Imagine that you can improve your life simply by creating more life in your eyes.

So far, the oldest person I've worked with was 101 years old. This patient experienced great changes and was able to see better and to improve his brain and eye functions quite a bit, even after just one session. Since he was one of only two patients over the age of a hundred with whom I have worked, I can only give these examples. I did, however, have success with both of them. I have also worked with several patients in their eighties and nineties and have witnessed tremendous positive changes in their visual systems through working with these exercises.

There is no doubt in my mind that, whether you are in your twenties, thirties, forties, fifties, sixties, seventies, or beyond, you can change the function of your eyes. There is enough elasticity in your brain to back it up. The problem isn't age itself, but whether or not a person is practicing the correct exercises for his or her age. It may be easier for a five-year-old child to get used to the weaker eye's workings by putting on a patch for four or eight hours a day as he or she plays. And truly, the brain has more plasticity when you're five than when you're seventy-five. But there are good, age-appropriate exercises you can do at anytime in your life that can change your visual system completely.

Chapter 2

Ten Steps to Better Vision

If you take care of your vision, not only will you see better, but you will also feel better, and you will positively affect your whole body's health. In addition to the exercises aimed at combating specific disorders and conditions, I have developed ten important steps that are perfect for incorporating into your daily life. These exercises are based on my seven principles of healthy vision:

1. Deep relaxation
2. Adjusting to light frequencies
3. Looking at details
4. Looking into the distance
5. Expanding your periphery
6. Balanced use of the two eyes
7. Body and eye coordination

These are the essential principles of healthy vision, and they can be attained by consistently practicing the eye exercises in this chapter.

Step 1: The Long Swing

I will never forget when I met Alan. He was a young French-Canadian banker who, while driving home after a meeting in his bank, fell asleep at the wheel and found himself in intensive care three days later. By the time he woke up, they had replaced his forehead with platinum. He had lost all his vision. The optic nerve in his left eye was destroyed, in addition to most of the optic nerve in his right eye. But that little bit of nerve tissue remained, so Alan discovered that he still had some visual sensation.

The physicians thought that only 4 percent of his potentially functional nerve was not enough to regain any vision. Alan heard about my book *The Handbook of Self Healing.* In it, I suggest that people who are legally blind start working with blinking lights in a dark room. Alan experimented with the techniques in the book, and, sure enough, the little bit of remaining optic nerve woke up. He called me in San Francisco and soon came out for a series of therapy sessions. Alan's girlfriend held his hand to walk him into the office because he couldn't see most objects. His brain did not yet know how to use that little bit of remaining healthy nerve tissue in his right eye.

During our first session we practiced an exercise called *the long swing.* As he did this exercise, he said, "I'm noticing twelve objects that I've never noticed before in the room." Within minutes, his sense of orientation built up even more. When the series of sessions finished, he no longer needed to be led around. The long swing is what is called an integrative exercise. It allowed Alan to perceive a sense of space.

The long swing exercise develops a sense of fluidity and flexibility that will allow you to look at details with more ease, to adapt to light easier, and to adapt to new, livelier visual habits.

How to Do the Long Swing

Stand with your legs slightly more than hip-width apart and your knees slightly bent. Hold your index finger about one foot in front of your face, pointing up to the ceiling. Look at your finger with a soft gaze. If you are legally blind, or even with correction have very poor vision, you can look at your index and middle fingers together. While looking at your finger(s), swing your body from side to side. As you swing to the right, twist your body so that your left heel rises slightly off the ground. As you twist your body to the left, your right heel raises slightly off the ground. If your hand becomes tired, you can switch hands. Do this at least twenty times.

You will notice the sensation that everything in the background seems to be moving in the opposite direction of your finger, like scenery passing by you as you look out the window of a train. Allow yourself to feel the sense of relaxation that comes when you don't need to place a hard focus on any one object. Move to the right, and the world moves to the left. Move to the left, and the world moves to the right.

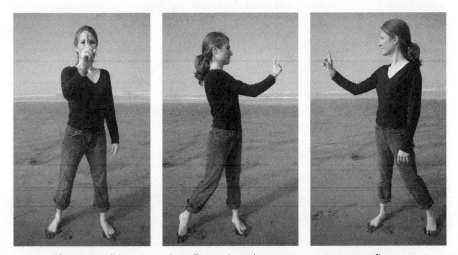

Figure 2.1. (a) Long swing, front view; keep your eye on your finger. (b) Long swing, right profile. (c) Long swing, left profile view.

Now hold your finger horizontally in front of your face. Move your finger up and down in front of you, moving your head vertically along with your finger. Remember to continue to hold a soft gaze. When you move up, everything in the background seems to be moving down. When you move down, everything seems to be moving up.

Next, hold your finger in front of you and do the long swing, pointing your finger to the ceiling as in the first explanation, but this time as you swing to one side, bend at the waist and sweep down in a half circle—just to knee level. Don't lower your head below your knees, but continue the swing until your arm is fully extended and you are looking up at your finger. This exercise should relax your eyes further.

The next step is very important. This is where we visualize the long swing. We close our eyes and do the movement with our bodies, and visualize in our mind's eye that the world is swinging back and forth, passing in front of our eyes. Everything you visualize is moving directly opposite. When you move to the right, the neighborhood moves to the left. When you move to the left, the whole world moves to the right. Remember how you saw objects this way. Now you open your eyes and continue the exercise.

When you look in this way, you stop yourself from freezing. It becomes easier to look at details and much easier to blink. Remind yourself to blink. Blinking will help you to relax.

When I started to work on my own vision, my eyes had a constant *nystagmus*, which is an involuntary rapid movement of the eyes caused by continuous strain from trying to see the world with a total lack of success. So I practiced the long swing for about forty minutes a day, and it immediately eased the involuntary flutter of my eyes. I had a feeling of more light entering my eyes. Details started to appear in the background, and when I started to look at details like windows and books on shelves, they gradually became clearer and clearer to me. Long swinging prepared my brain for new exercises.

When you practice the rest of the exercises in this book followed by long swinging, you will absorb the exercises better because long swinging alleviates tension and stiffness in the brain, in addition to preparing us to learn and benefit from new visual techniques.

I will never forget the time when I was walking in the streets of Tel Aviv with my eye instructor, Jacob, who was then only sixteen years old. Jacob told me to look at a building full of windows. In the corners of the windows I could see tiny, fuzzy black squares, which I later realized were air conditioners. At Jacob's instruction, I looked from window to air conditioner, back and forth for a whole summer, not understanding why I was doing this. Slowly, by looking at windows and air conditioners, looking at patterns of squares, a new habit developed in me, a habit of looking and not freezing. Long swinging helped to prepare me for this exercise and alleviated the rigidity that prevented me from looking at details, which allowed the program to sink in.

The reason that long swinging is referred to as an integrative exercise is that it takes you away from the stress you're used to. When people wear thick glasses that have a very specific focal point, they often strain their eyes so much that it becomes very difficult for them to look with vitality at the world. They look without seeing details, partially from fatigue and partially from the habits they have developed by straining to see. Long swinging breaks that tension. You cannot stare with this exercise, so more light enters your eyes through the movement, and therefore you won't need to strain to bring the new programming to your brain.

The long swinging exercise will also help you to develop your peripheral vision and to create a better sense of orientation. You don't have to swing for forty minutes at a time. In fact, even two minutes of twenty swings can help you loosen up. Think of it as warming up before a workout.

Step 2: Looking into the Distance

It is no coincidence that our school is located near the beach. In fact, it took us almost five years to convince San Francisco authorities and neighborhood groups to allow us to operate in this residential area. The reason this location is ideal for us is that we look at the waves on a daily basis and use their sparkling beauty in our work. They shine in sunlight and have different coloration, even in the fog. You can almost always see waves here, even when the weather is gray.

Look at the waves. Look at the sky. Look at the clouds. Look at the hills and valleys.

If you are not near the beach, look out your window at the many other buildings.

When you look near (as when staring at a computer screen), you unknowingly strain your eyes. The *ciliary* muscles contract, and this changes the shape of your lens from flat to round. When you look into the distance, however, the ciliary muscles relax, and the suspensory ligaments keep the lens flat and more flexible.

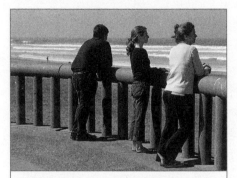

Figure 2.2. The reason this location is ideal for us is that we look at the waves on a daily basis and use their sparkling beauty in our work.

Many people in our culture are used to eyestrain from looking at computers, televisions, and books so much of the time. They pay attention to the contents and not to their eyes, which causes them to strain. Looking close makes you strain. Looking with boredom makes you strain. When you push on with the computer project, or the television show, or the book, you strain your eyes—even when you are aware of the strain.

Pay attention so that your face is relaxed and your jaw is not clenched. Release and rest your eyes. If it is possible, give yourself a few hours away from close work. Even if it is a deadline you are struggling to meet, do yourself a favor and take ten minutes to rest your eyes by looking into the distance. Look at the movements of the waves or the clouds. *Look into the distance.*

Never look closer than forty yards away, because you need to look far enough to rest the eyes from looking near. Know that when you look into the distance, you don't have to stay focused on one point; you can scan or look at different areas within the point you are looking at. Remember to blink and to avoid straining to see it. If it is fuzzy, let it be fuzzy.

For at least ten minutes every single day, look into the distance. If you wear corrective lenses, be brave: take your contact lenses out, take your glasses off, and allow your eyes to enjoy a breath of fresh air. One student in San Francisco came to me and said that after two and a half weeks of not wearing her lenses, she had started to feel comfortable, because of "the air bouncing on her eyes." This habit will reduce your dependency on glasses or lenses, and it will gradually strengthen your visual system.

Looking into the Distance Can Help to Prevent Cataracts!

If you can share this simple concept with other people, you will help to create a revolution in the world by helping to prevent the otherwise predictable cataract. Today, most physicians believe that, sooner or later, most people will develop cataracts. Looking into the distance can prevent the onset of cataracts because it gives the lens its full mobility and more life.

I realize that even if you practice this exercise every day, you will probably not look into the distance as much as life requires you to look near. Nevertheless, looking into the distance for eight to ten minutes, three times a day, will at least allow your eyes to rest and will compensate for the strain of looking near.

Step 3: Exploring the Periphery

It is impossible to strain your eyes while looking centrally if you remember to simultaneously focus on your periphery. In our culture, we suppress parts of the eye that help us to see well naturally. It is a subconscious suppression. We suppress the periphery because we make it irrelevant to our lives. As we focus on objects in front of us,

Discovering Your Strong Eye

About 20 percent of the people that I've met have no difference in strength between their two eyes. Even so, the majority of people do have very different levels of strength between their eyes. A small number of those people have one eye stronger for looking from a distance, and the other is stronger for looking near.

If you experience an extreme difference of ability between your two eyes, you probably already know it by now. You may know which eye needs a stronger prescription for correction. You may have had an injury to one of your eyes, or you may simply be aware of which eye you tend to use to look. If you are not sure which one of your eyes is your dominant eye, there is a way you can test it.

To see which eye is dominant for distance, make a loose fist with a pencil-sized hole through the center, like a telescope. Hold your loose fist about a foot away from your face. (It could be closer for people who see poorly or farther for people who see sharply.) With both eyes at the same time, look at some distant point through the hole in your fist. Now close one eye and see if that point disappears. For example, if your stronger eye is your left eye, when you close the right eye, you will still see the object through your fist. When you close the left eye, you will not see the object, and vice versa. Then you'll know which eye is stronger.

To see which eye is dominant for close distances, look at a page in this book, with its big and small letters. Look at the smallest letters you can see, and then close one eye at a time. Whichever eye can see the small letters better is your strong eye for nearby vision.

If you cannot figure out on your own which eye is stronger, you can go to an optometrist and ask for help.

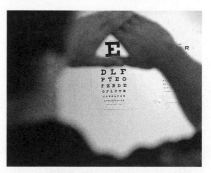

Figure 2.3. Discovering the dominant eye.

we simply don't pay attention to what's around us. On the other hand, our ancient fathers and mothers, our predecessors, had to pay attention to their surroundings; in the jungle, you wouldn't last more than a week without noticing the periphery. In fact, you would be eaten or you would starve to death if you didn't notice what was around you.

But we ignore the periphery so we can focus on computers and paperwork all day without being distracted by our environment. We try to concentrate on the task at hand and can't be distracted by the commotions around us. When we don't notice the periphery, the strain on our central vision becomes much greater, which, in time, makes us use it poorly. This causes us to strain our central vision, decreasing its clarity and eventually losing it. The old adage that says use it or lose it holds true here. With time, we lose the connection between our brain, our optic nerve, and the rod cells of the periphery. Along with genetic tendencies, this can be a cause of glaucoma.

What we need to do right now is to exercise our periphery.

Periphery Exercise 1: Look into the Distance

Sit somewhere comfortable where you can see something in the distance that you enjoy looking at. As you look into the distance, start to wave your hands to the sides of your head to notify your eyes that a periphery exists. Don't look at your hands waving; just look into the distance. Allow your eyes to recognize the movement of your hands.

Wave your hands in such a way that your fingers point toward you and your wrists are

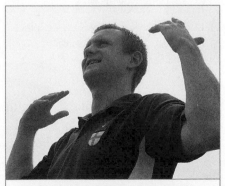

Figure 2.4. Will wakes up his periphery with a wave of his hands as he looks at the distance.

loose. Do this for a minute or two. As you do this, you should feel your eyes release their tension; this relaxation in your eyes is vitally important to healthy vision.

Periphery Exercise 2: The Small Pieces of Paper

Cut out a small piece of opaque paper (about one inch by two inches) and tape the paper horizontally on the bridge of your nose so that the wide parts are centered in front of your eyes. This will disrupt part of your vision.

Walk around in a familiar environment with this paper on your nose for a minute or two. Now sit down and wave your hands to the sides of your head like you did before. Stand up and sit down several times, moving your whole body up and down, as you wave your hands to the sides. As you do this, it reveals to your brain the existence of a moving periphery with which it normally does not connect.

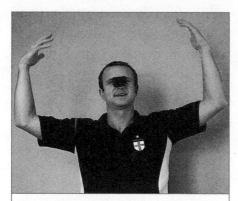

Figure 2.5. Will uses the smallest piece of paper to block his central vision while activating his periphery.

In the past, people used to walk at night, sometimes in total darkness and sometimes with light from the stars and moon. Imagine how important it was for them to notice things moving in their periphery at night! For millions of years, our ancestors used to walk this way. Now we have the city lights at night, and our peripheral cells are hardly being used because they are mainly designed for night vision.

Waving our hands to our sides wakes up the peripheral cells because the rods of the retina respond to movement rather than to still images; conversely, the cones respond better to a still picture. These

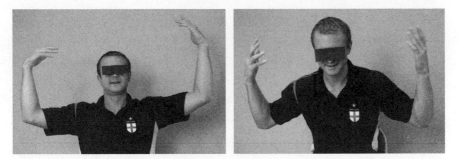

Figure 2.6. (a) Will blocks even more of his central vision. (b) As he waves, he leans forward and back to create more movement in his periphery.

cones are mainly in the central part of the retina (the macula) and are used to look at details. An overwhelming number of the retina's cells are the rods, which respond mainly to the impression of movement. When we exercise these rods, we take away a lot of stress from the overworked cones, and we make it easier for them to function more correctly. Instead of the brain forcing the eye to freeze and to strenuously see a picture, the brain will command the eye to look gently and easily in order to see the entire landscape better.

Next, put a longer piece of paper (one inch by five inches) on the bridge of your nose and repeat this exercise. Then use a piece of paper that is one inch by seven inches. By blocking so much of your central vision, and even some of your peripheral vision, you will discover a periphery that you hardly ever use consciously. Now go back to the medium-sized paper and repeat the exercise. Then use the small piece of paper and repeat the exercise for a final time. You may find that the small piece now seems even smaller in your perception. That is because much of your brain that had been suppressed is now engaged in peripheral vision.

To finish, take the small paper off, stand, and do the long swing so your brain will absorb the exercise you have just performed.

Step 4: Sunning and Skying

Sunning

Surrendering to the sun briefly each day can make a huge difference in terms of our overall feeling of well-being.

Since the 1980s, physicians have warned us against the dangers of exposure to the sun. Now they understand the benefits of sunlight and recommend that we have some exposure to it daily. The sun is one of the best nurturers that nature has given us. It is important, however, to adapt your eyes to the strong light of the sun. Sunning is a great exercise for this purpose because it is relaxing to the eyes and can also help you with your sleep.

I once had a patient who complained about terrible insomnia. She had not slept for many nights and had a tremendous amount of tension. I taught her the sunning exercise and massaged her in the sun. After her first session, she went home and slept right through the night; after taking only three sessions at the school, she reported that she had slept much better. That was years ago. To this day, she practices the sunning technique and no longer experiences sleep deprivation.

Today, physicians suggest that we should not expose ourselves to the sun, except before 10 a.m. and after 5 p.m. In my opinion, we should sometimes expose ourselves to the sun even at midday. If you are sensitive to sunlight, you should start by practicing the sunning exercise early in the morning or near dusk, or for just five minutes at a time in the middle of the day.

To begin sunning, all you need to do is close your eyes and face the sun. Now move your head from side to side, rotating it from shoulder to shoulder. As you face the sun, the sphincter pupillae constrict the pupils. As you move your head away toward one shoulder, the radial dilator muscle dilates the pupil, even though your eyes are closed. Some people find it easy to move their head 180 degrees from shoulder to shoulder. If you find this full range of motion difficult,

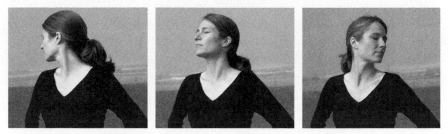

Figure 2.7. (a) Move your head from side to side,
rotating it from shoulder to shoulder. (b) As you face the sun,
the sphincter pupillae constrict the pupils even with the eyes closed.
(c) Move your opposite shoulder slightly forward if your neck
does not move as freely as this yoga student.

simply bring your opposite shoulder forward slightly; it will help you to move your head all the way toward the side and to compensate for the limited range of motion until you loosen up. The more you practice this exercise, the more your range of motion and flexibility will increase.

The movements should not be fast, but they should not be slow, either. Just relax, breathe deeply and slowly, and visualize that the sun, with its energy and light, is penetrating your face and nurturing your eyes as well as your mind. Your eyelids should be closed softly; don't squeeze your eyelids shut. You want the eyelids to close as gently as if you were about to go to sleep. The less you squeeze your eyelids, the more relaxed your eyes will become.

When I was in high school, I had been doing this sunning exercise on a camping trip. Seeing me rotate my head back and forth, a girl asked, "Why do you keep saying no? Can't you say yes?" So I moved my head up and down as if to nod "yes," and I had a revelation. I noticed that this movement led to a greater variability in the angles at which light reached my eyes, thus awakening more parts of them. This additional exercise allowed for greater stimulation and an increased sensation of lightness and darkness. I would recommend that this additional exercise be included during sunning.

Whenever you experience that difference between extremes of dark and light, your pupils become stronger. The pupils of most modern people are very weak because they wear sunglasses when they're outside, which weakens the pupils. Automatic activities, like those of the eye's iris muscles that affect the pupils, are influenced by function and use. The more you constrict and expand your pupils, the stronger the iris muscles become. Your retina also benefits from more concentrated light, and blood flows much better to the eye as a result of the pupils contracting and expanding.

The sunning exercise is mandatory for people who want to improve their vision. Like any exercise, it doesn't create drastic change for everyone. But quite a few of my clients have experienced huge vision improvement and have reduced the strength of their eyeglass prescriptions when they have diligently practiced sunning. When you have a break at work or school, I recommend sunning instead of smoking cigarettes or drinking coffee.

Skying

Skying is a simple exercise. It is similar to sunning, but you do this as an alternative when there is no sun. You just put one hand behind the back of your head and one hand on your forehead, applying pressure so that you massage your head as you turn it from side to side. Now move your head from side to side like you are sunning and blink rapidly at the sky.

After two minutes of skying, do a minute of swinging. Then do three minutes of skying and two minutes of swinging. Then do three more minutes of skying

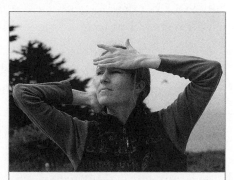

Figure 2.8. Apply great pressure to the head, holding the arms fixed as you blink at the sky and turn only your head from side to side.

and two more minutes of swinging. This is an antisquinting exercise, and as you sky and then swing, you are letting more light into your eyes and stopping the tendency to squint.

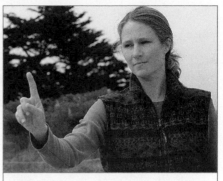

Figure 2.9. Long swinging and skying go hand in hand.

Step 5: Night Walking

Night walking is the complementary exercise to sunning. The idea is simply to walk at night, in the dark, with only the light of the moon and the stars to guide your way.

Most of us, even if we live outside of a city, are surrounded by the glow of city lights. Those of us who live in remote areas often use flashlights. We have all learned to live with artificial lights, but once you get completely away from them for a time, you begin to realize how profoundly the city lights burden your eyes. Yes, we are happy to have them because they light the streets, making us safer and allowing for activity after the sun has fallen. But remember, as valuable as they may be to our industry and safety, this constant light is not beneficial to our eyes. For this reason, we must take part in exercises (like night walking) that strengthen our eyes and compensate for the burden of city lights.

Every time I teach an extensive eye course, we spend one evening in which we walk together in the dark. It is very pleasant for all of us to walk in places like the park, where we are free from artificial light. Of course, it can be dangerous to walk in the dark whether you live in the city or in the country, so I recommend that, when practicing night walking, you get a group of friends to walk together.

In the dark of night, it takes only three to four minutes to expand your pupils to nine times their normal size in the daytime. It takes about forty minutes to wake up the rods of the retina that sense movement and periphery. After night walking for about fifty minutes, you are finally utilizing the full potential of your eyes.

Night walking is a wonderful opportunity to try all the other exercises you are learning. After finding a nice, safe place to walk in the dark, set out and explore the many benefits of this practice. During your walk, stop at times and do the long swing exercise. Allow yourself the time to adjust to the darkness, and let your brain comprehend the change it is experiencing.

Palming (discussed in the next section) is another exercise that works great as an addition to night walking because it allows your eyes to better adjust to the dark. After they have properly adjusted, you can try peripheral exercises if you feel secure in your surroundings. Tape a short piece of paper between your eyes, and wave your hands to the sides of your head while walking to wake up the periphery.

By the time you finish your night walking, you will have awakened your eyes and reminded your brain of the way it used to function in a more primitive time, before light pollution filled the earth. Therefore, if you are serious about improving your eyes, night walking is an effective and enjoyable exercise that I would recommend doing at least twice a month when weather permits.

Step 6: Palming

Note: Before palming, individuals with glaucoma should read "Special Instructions for Palming with Glaucoma" in Chapter 6 for important modifications to this exercise.

Tibetan Yogis have been practicing palming for more than 1,500 years. It is an exercise that complements every other practice you will learn from this book.

Many people believe that they receive sufficient rest for their eyes while they are asleep. While sleep is very important, even with adequate sleep, many people still experience eye fatigue. There are a few reasons why this happens. One reason is that in these modern times we often hear noise around us while we are asleep; even though we don't feel disturbed, the noise upsets our rest on a subconscious level. The other reason sleep often fails to sufficiently rest our eyes is that many people sleep in rooms that are not completely dark. I suggest that you darken your bedroom as much as you can. The darker the room, the more rest you will give your eyes. Sleeping in total darkness produces hormones, such as melatonin, that relax your body, allowing you to experience deeper and more refreshing sleep.

In order for sleep to be completely satisfying, quite often we dream. Dreams enhance our state of being; it is as though they wash away the day. Although dreams allow for physical and mental relaxation, the saccadic movement during dreams doesn't allow for full relaxation of the eyes.

The greatest rest is a conscious rest, not a passive rest. William Bates, the originator of eye exercises in the modern world, understood this principle. And the Tibetan Yogis, who have mastered the art of meditation, understand this concept perhaps even better than anyone else. When you meditate, you enter a state of transcendental relaxation. As with meditation, palming helps us to quiet the mind and focus on eye relaxation. This produces a very powerful effect.

There is a great Jewish adage that says the truth is always simple. The way to the truth, however, may be complex.

To palm correctly, and to receive the benefits of this powerful exercise, you first have to engage in the correct preparation. You must have relaxed hands because this exercise takes you to a place where your hands nurture your eyes. Healthy hands can bring warmth, energy, and blood flow to the eyes, but there is no way for you to energize your eyes if your hands are angry, irritated, or numb in any way. Ensuring relaxed hands is necessary to receive benefits from this exercise.

Preparing to Palm

The most important thing when palming is that you are not stressed. I recommend massaging your temples, face, shoulders, and the top of your head in order to bring good blood flow to the eyes and become as relaxed as possible.

Loosen your shoulders. Move your shoulders together in a rotating motion, forward and then back. Then rotate each shoulder separately,

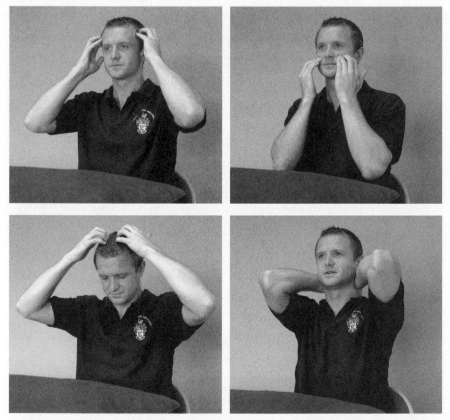

Figure 2.10. (a) Massage the scalp and temple. (b) Massage the cheek bones. (c) Massage the scalp. (d) Massage the neck.

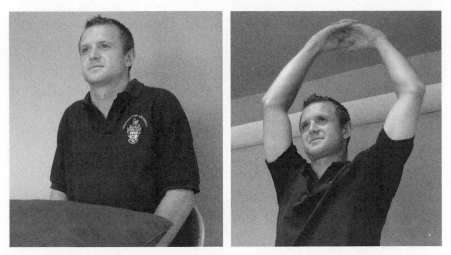

Figure 2.11. (a) Move your shoulders together in a rotating motion, forward and then back. (b) Intertwine your fingers, straighten your arms, and move your arms in a circular motion.

forward and back. Picture that the shoulder tip is moving the shoulder. Now tap on the tip of the shoulder with your opposite hand and say out loud, "Shoulder tip." Moving the shoulders in a rotating motion increases blood circulation; as you repeat this exercise several times, your shoulders will feel lighter.

Next, lift your arm up and move your whole arm in a rotating motion, imagining that your fingertips are moving your arm. By focusing on your fingertips, your body will naturally loosen. Tap the wall with your fingertips and say, "Fingertips." Then put your opposite hand on your shoulder and move it in a rotating motion. Repeat this series of movements with the opposite shoulder and hand.

Quite often the area between the shoulders gets contracted, and energy becomes trapped because there is not enough movement happening in that area. Consequently, there is not enough blood flow, which quite literally freezes the hands.

The next step for palming is to open and close your fingers one hundred times, visualizing that the fingertips are initiating the movement.

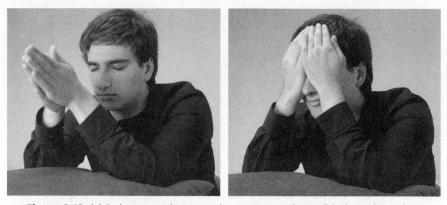

Figure 2.12. (a) Rub your palms together to warm them. (b) Place the palms very gently over the eye orbits, putting no pressure on the face.

From time to time, tap with your fingertips on the opposite forearm. Now massage your hands, front and back, by pretending you are washing them with soap and water. Then rub your two palms together, with the front of your fingers rubbing back and forth against each other in a circular motion.

The result of this exercise is that your fingers will be warm and your hands will be loose. The warmth and relaxation of your hands will enable you now to palm in a way that is correct and beneficial. Though it is very important to be relaxed while palming, not all these shoulder exercises will be necessary each time. At the very least, rub your palms together to warm them; then intertwine your fingers, straighten your arms, and move your arms in a circular motion. Utilize your full range of motion several times in both directions, first with your hands palm to palm, and then with your palms facing outward. Depending on the time available, these relaxation exercises may last anywhere between two to eight minutes.

How to Palm

Now that you have prepared your body for palming, sit somewhere comfortable. You need to have your elbows resting on pillows or on a table top with a pillow so that your head is leaning neither forward nor backward. In other words, you are sitting comfortably in good posture. It is very important that you are not holding your arms up, that you are not straining your neck by letting your head tilt back, and, most important, that *you never put any pressure on your face at all.* If you put your weight on anything, it is on your elbows. Rub your palms together to warm them and place them very gently over the eye orbits. The palms never touch the eyelids, but notice how your palms feel *over* your eye lids, over the entire eye orbit. Can you feel the warmth? Do your hands feel nurturing as they sit ever so lightly over your eye orbits? This is important. If you are stressed or angry, your palming session will not feel good. Repeat the exercises to prepare for palming or do some kind of activity that helps you to let go of the stress or the anger you are carrying.

How Long Should You Palm?

The duration of your palming may change depending on your schedule and your state of mind. If you are busy, perhaps you might take a break in the middle of your work from time to time and sit for a few minutes to palm. You can palm for one minute just to rest the eyes, but it takes a minimum of six minutes to clear the retina from neurological waste products. Of course, it is even more wonderful if you can palm for fifteen or twenty minutes at a time!

Visualization While Palming

While you palm, there are two visualizations that will help you to receive the full benefit of this exercise. The first is that you visualize a figure eight, or an infinity sign. You can visualize a boat on the ocean moving in the figure-eight pattern, or a train in the mountains traveling a route shaped like an infinity sign. This is a fluid movement that helps your mind be able to travel from detail to detail easily and fluidly.

The second visualization is of total blackness and increasing blackness. Close your eyes and begin palming. Now visualize that the room you are in is being painted black. Visualize that your body is being painted black. Visualize that the neighborhood is being painted black. Visualize that the city is being painted black. Visualize black paint covering the entire world. Visualize that all the stars and the sun are being painted black. This is total blackness you are visualizing. Black is the color that allows the optic nerve to relax.

Breathing While Palming

Remember to inhale and exhale slowly while palming. Visualize your abdomen rising slowly and falling gently. Count to eight as you slowly breathe in, then count to eleven as you slowly breathe out. Don't tense up; just let yourself breathe in and out.

Right now, you feel that your whole upper torso is expanding while you inhale and shrinking as you exhale. At the same time, you should feel that your head expands as you inhale and shrinks as you exhale. You visualize that your pelvis expands as you inhale and shrinks as you exhale, or that your legs expand as you breathe in and shrink as you breathe out. You visualize that your whole body expands as you breathe in and shrinks as you breathe out.

Relaxing the Ears

A good addition to palming the eyes is resting the ears from external noise. As a result of the noise we live in, our senses are under continuous pressure. Pressure causes tension, and if we are tense, we can never get to a place of relaxed eyes.

So, when you finish palming, rub your hands together again to increase the blood flow to your fingers; then put your thumbs deep inside your ears. Listen to your breath. What does it sound like? It may sound like ocean waves or wind. Breathe deeply and slowly to the count of ten, and palm again. You will feel your neck muscles becoming loose, and your whole head will start to relax.

Benefits of Palming

People who have multiple sclerosis and have an attack on their visual system quite often receive cortisone treatments from their doctors. In many cases, if such patients just sat down for a whole day palming with a nice cloth around their eyes, they would be able to overcome the attack on their visual system simply through rest. It's a simple truth that relaxation is very powerful. When you relax completely, your body returns to its highest and best functioning.

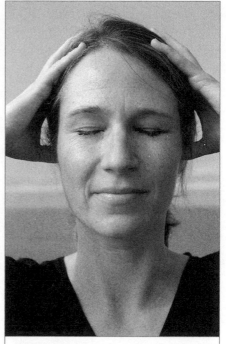

Figure 2.13. Put your thumbs deep inside your ears. Listen to your breath.

I am in awe of nature for giving us such wonderful tools with which to see. In all its complexity, nature has fine-tuned our vision. Vision is completely integrated with our development as human beings and is progressing side by side with it. Most of the visual process is subconscious and unknown to us. But science is gradually realizing the marvelous energy behind vision!

We have 125 million photoreceptor cells in each retina, with a billion light rays bouncing against some of them every single minute, converting light into visual energy. To allow the process to function at its best, we need to learn not to squint. You may not be aware that your eyes squint even when you sleep and dream.

Palming can work away our tendency to squint. When you palm with soft, relaxed hands, and when you see black, there is a wonderful release of the eyelids, the temples, the forehead, and the entire skull. Squinting is eliminated, and you notice a relaxed sensation as you open your eyes. You also sense much more periphery because, with fully open eyelids, much more light can penetrate your eyes.

Quite often, physicians say that squinting does not have any ill effects, but it does. In this respect, the wisdom of the Tibetan Yogis was definitely greater than the wisdom of modern medicine. Modern medicine still needs to adopt the concept that rest and relaxation are so powerful.

Combining Palming with Other Exercises

After you have mastered palming, next time you are sunning, practicing the long swing, or night walking, stop for a few moments, put your hands over your eye orbits, and do your palming. Breathe slowly, in deep breaths. Your pupils will have time to enlarge a bit. Then take your hands off and return to your other exercise.

From time to time, also stop to massage your eyebrows. Massage the right eyebrow from the bridge of your nose to your temple; then do the same thing on the left side. Massage your cheekbones and stretch the muscles of your cheekbones from nose to ear. Every time you firmly massage your cheekbone, you may find that more light penetrates your eyes and you experience a sense of less squinting.

Step 7: Shifting

Shifting is an exercise designed to wake up your macula and help to develop the retina. In the retina, we have 125 million photoreceptors. Five million of them look at fine details, and 120 million of them look at the general picture. When we try to look at fine details, we can see them well only if we look at them centrally. We see them poorly, however, if we try to see them with our peripheral vision.

Shifting is all about moving your gaze from detail to detail. The eye

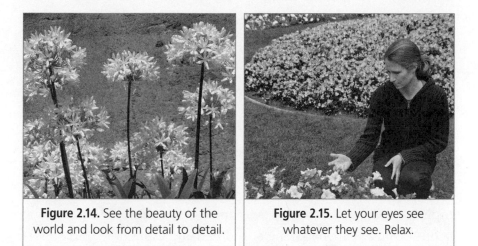

Figure 2.14. See the beauty of the world and look from detail to detail.

Figure 2.15. Let your eyes see whatever they see. Relax.

has a natural tendency to shift from point to point. If you are the type of person who takes your time to see the beauty of the world and to look from detail to detail, you've already started this exercise.

Practicing Shifting

All you need to do is to open your eyes and look at details, without contacts and without glasses. The beauty of this exercise, and the reason you can feel good about practicing it without glasses, is that you don't need to strain to try and see details clearly or perfectly. You just observe them. Let your eyes see whatever they see. Relax. If what you see is clear, that is wonderful. If what you see is fuzzy, that is wonderful, too! So enjoy the clarity or relax and maybe start to enjoy the fuzziness.

After you observe the details of whatever you are looking at, close your eyes and visualize the margins and distances between details. Think about the contrast between those details. Have you ever thought about the pleasure of seeing contrast? Even if your general vision is fuzzy, when you notice the contrast between details, you start to activate the mechanism of perception that is so important when trying to establish a visual sense of your environment.

You can look at details from near, or you can look at details from afar. Go for a walk and look at a house. Then look down at the sidewalk. Look at a road and then look at another house. From time to time, look into the distance for a short moment; then look back at the details of the street, the details of the road, and the details of the houses. Embrace the contrast.

Some people think the normal speed of the macula is as quick as seventy-two eye movements per second. The macula moves at a great speed, and we want to help our eyes look from detail to detail rapidly, by doing it correctly and looking right. By shifting, looking at one detail and then looking at another, and examining the contrast between these details, we can reverse this habit and open up the tendency to truly look.

Look at More Details

Now that you are slowing down to notice the details of your environment, you can further vitalize your eyes by looking at even smaller and smaller details.

There was a time when I looked at details for thirteen hours a day, every day. I looked at windows and air conditioners. I looked at blinds and bricks. I would sometimes ask a friend of mine with better vision to look at the exact details that I was looking at and to describe them to me. My friend would always describe different details than the ones I saw, and this would make me want to study the details even more.

It is also helpful to get a group of people to stand and look at details together. As the group looks at an environment, such as the waves on the ocean, they take turns describing what they see. Someone might describe a boat or a ship at a distance. Someone else might describe the boat's shape or color even more specifically. There could be a particular light in the horizon with different coloration. The larger the number of people describing these details, the more everyone can find new things to look for and discover new ways of seeing.

This happens instinctively with little kids because they get so excited when they respond to something they see. The same thing is true for us adults: the more we look at details, the more stimulated we get. That sense of excitement in our eyes is apparent, and when anyone looks at our eyes, they see vitality in them. There is nothing as frozen as eyes that don't look, and there is nothing as alive as eyes that do look. When you look from point to point, you project that you have a sense of presence and attention.

The pleasure of looking at details is a form of unity with the world that nature gave us. The more we look on a regular basis, the less casual life is for us. Everything in life becomes interesting as we see all the differentiation within it.

I remember a biker who came to one of my classes in the 1980s. He rode his motorcycle from the Peninsula, a forty-minute ride to our school. After studying for two and a half hours in a vision class, he went straight to Golden Gate Park just to watch the beautiful flowers in the Arboretum, one by one. He looked at their petals and at their veins. He looked at their stems and at their leaves. Smaller and smaller details he continued to find. The class had stimulated him to want to look at beauty.

I used to ask my daughter, Adar, to go to the beach with me. I would take along an eye chart, some tennis balls, and her glasses, which had an obstruction for her left eye—it was her stronger eye—to give her right eye a chance to work more. Since she almost always resisted going, I had to tempt her by suggesting that I would put her on my shoulders. Fortunately, she remembered that she had enjoyed being on my shoulders from the time she was a baby, so she would agree. When we arrived at the beach, she would do eye exercises as she looked at the waves and into the distance. Eventually, Adar began to notice that her reading of the chart had become much better and would always say, "Daddy, why did I oppose coming to the beach? It's just so nice to be here."

On our way to the beach we would stop from time to time, and I'd get her to look at signs. At times, we would stop at a flowerbed right near the beach, and I'd ask her to count two hundred petals with her weak right eye. As she counted, I would look at my watch and find the count had taken between fifty-five and fifty-nine seconds. This always surprised me because it seemed too quick. I also remember another time during her adolescence, while massaging and relaxing her in a dark room, I asked, "Adar, how many petals can you count in one minute?"

She answered that she could count between thirty-five and forty.

So I said, "Adar, I have timed you and found that you can count two hundred of them in less than one minute."

Upon that, she replied, "But, Daddy, I can't follow my count."

"That is the exact point," I answered. "What happened was that you had counted automatically, and by exceeding normal speed with your counting, you engaged the macula in a function it already knows how to perform. You directed your macula to look."

So, my daughter, whose lens was removed, and whose cornea is small, was able to exceed all expectations about her vision by connecting her brain and her macula. Everyone can do the same, either with a healthy eye or with an eye that has some defect. Like my daughter, you too can make the connection between your brain and your macula. You can move from detail to detail rapidly, and as a result your vision can become as sharp as my daughter's vision had.

Find a lovely place to sit and look at beauty, to look from detail to detail of a beautiful thing. Once you gain this desire, the world will look beautiful to you, and you will want to mobilize yourself. It is so important that you retain curiosity about details. As children, we have it naturally; as adults, we have to make an effort to give it our attention and our souls. It is wrong to be childish, because that is immature and taxes you, but it is wonderful to be childlike, to be unfrozen and in a state of perpetual awe.

If you were born with macular degeneration or have an inclination toward it, looking at details will slow it down and may even reverse it. Looking from detail to detail is the work of the macula. Your macula becomes activated as many millions of cells start to come alive; their activity triggers activity in the brain. This activity in turn creates more synapses between

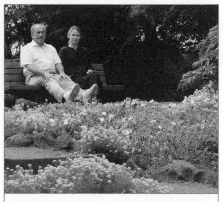

Figure 2.16. Find a lovely place to sit and look at beauty.

the macula and the brain, and between the brain and the macula. It's amazing how a small part of our body, the macula of the eye, can energize the whole body. It's also important that all of us strengthen our macula so we will be able to see well for the hundred or more years that we could live.

Shifting is one of the best habits to get into.

Read the Fine Print

People used to look at raindrops on leaves. They used to look at fruit that matured on the tops of trees. Nowadays, people tend to look just at the big picture. We learn to try and look at whole paragraphs of pages, just to grab their contents without looking at details.

In the past, we used to revere the written word. We used to read poetry. People used to look at every word and find something to respect. People used to read the same poem over and over again and find new meaning each new time they read it. Those times are over. These days, every poet who would try to live off poetry may just as well apply for welfare because there's no way that he or she can make enough money by selling it. On the other end, suspense stories and prose with low-level content sell, and because they're not extremely interesting when you look at them page by page, people don't mind skimming through a whole novel to get the gist of it. This only weakens the activity of the macula. It's the tragedy of the modern world that we don't really engage with great presence in whatever we're looking at.

This next exercise, therefore, is a good push in the opposite direction. Look at the page in this book with different sized paragraphs of print. Look at the third print size, which is the size of normal print.

No one has perfect vision all the time, and our eyesight varies.

Figure 2.17. Look at each letter slowly, in detail, as if you were writing it with your mind.

Bates checked hundreds of thou-sands of eyes

human and animal, young and old.

While his subjects slept, ate, got sick, underwent anesthesia,

posed for photos, did arithmetic, gazed at stars, played ball, and sewed on buttons,

Bates tagged after them and measured their vision.

The results surprised him.

Bad vision got worse, got a little better, had flashes of perfect vision.

Sleep often produced worse vision.

Normal eyes went nearsighted every time the subject told a lie.

Look at each letter slowly, in detail, as if you were writing it with your mind. Follow each part of each letter with your eyes, point by point, line by line. For example, if you see a Z, you can look at the lower line of the letter; then notice the middle line, and gradually take in the top line. Look even closer to see many different points in the bottom line, many points in the middle line, and many points in the upper line. Try to distinguish between parts of the Z, even though it is just one letter. Then continue to look at all the other different letters in this same way. Look at each different part of each letter as if you were writing them slowly with dark ink

This way of looking utilizes the macula, the center of the retina, in the exact way you looked at the details in the world when you were an infant. At first, you may not have seen them well. But once you looked at whichever details you could see, you woke up the connection between the brain and the macula.

Now look at the first print size: the large print. Look from point to point on each letter in the large print. Then look back at the smaller print size and find whether you see them better than before. You can do this same exercise from two perspectives. You can start with small print and then look at larger print, or vice versa. In both ways, you should be able to reach the same results. You are training your brain to look at smaller areas than your normal tendency.

After you read the print in this way, look away from the page for a minute and see if you remember what you read. It is amazing how many people have absolutely no recollection of the text, or a very limited recollection.

I enjoy sharing this story about someone in a recent class who lost vision in one eye almost completely and could not really see text. I had him read an eye chart, and he could read only eight letters. When I quickly moved his face away from the chart, he did not remember even one out of those eight letters, for three times in a row. We finally made some progress when he remembered at least one. Consequently, he started to have some vision in an eye that both he and his doctors had dismissed as being completely blind. The first day of the class, he had to be led around by another person; that was when his stronger eye, or what he called his "seeing eye," was patched. The second day, he still had to be led around but felt more confident and could not be stopped. After trying to recollect what was on the chart, he walked with an eye patch without any disturbance and looked with the eye that he had dismissed as blind. He didn't see well yet, but he was not blind.

On a much smaller scale, what's amazing is when you start to remember part of what you read; even if you don't remember but just try to recollect it, you'll find that the vision in both eyes becomes much stronger.

This work with the macula can change you physically and spiritually. Quite often, we have a single-minded idea about the reality of life, when the reality of life actually has many levels and many variations. Looking at many details helps you experience the variations that both the physical and the psychological worlds have to offer.

The Ink Is Black and the Page Is White

With a small piece of paper taped to the bridge of your nose to block the central vision in your strong eye, look at an eye chart in bright sunlight or under bright inside light. Look at the page and imagine that the black ink of the print is interrupting the white of the page. Slowly move your attention from letter to letter. Start with the large print in line one. Meanwhile, wave your hand to the side of the stronger eye. This way you're simultaneously working to increase the periphery of the stronger eye and improving the central vision of the weaker eye.

You are engaging your weaker eye in practice that it's not used to. Normally, the strong eye dominates. When there is stress on the visual system—and I would like to suggest that most of us, even those who have good vision, have some visual stress—the tendency of the system is to use the strong parts and suppress the weak ones.

But this is unhealthy for us. It makes us work very hard to see. When you wave to the side of the strong eye and look with the weaker eye, you wake up cells in the eye and in the brain that normally are not working. When you wake them up, there's a great relief because there is more balance in the system, and no one group of cells works harder than the others.

Now close your eyes and imagine that the space is white and the ink is black, and remember a single letter you just saw. It will give you a sense that you are really looking at that letter. Say out loud, "The ink is black and the page is white." You don't need to wave your hand while your eyes are closed, but you can imagine that you are waving your hand to the side of the strong eye while reading with the weaker eye. Then open your eyes and wave to the side of the strong eye and read the next line with the weaker eye. Now close your eyes and say out loud, three times, "The ink is black and the page is white." Then open your eyes and wave your hand to the side and read the next line. Next, look away into the distance, and wave your hand to the side of your head. Now look back at the fourth line without changing the distance at which you started; then close your eyes and visualize the letters again. Repeat the process for the last lines of text. Each time you close your eyes, say out loud, "The ink is black and the page is white." Or say the opposite: "The page is white and the ink is black."

When you finish doing all these movements, look back at the third line and see how clear it became. Then look back at line number one. What you did is that you trained your brain to look at smaller details with the eye that normally did not work as much as the other. In this way, you create equality in your brain, which takes away the stress from underusing the weaker eye and overusing the stronger eye.

You should see these results rather quickly. Most people are astounded at how much better they can see when they take the paper away from their eyes. For a time span that could last for two seconds to several minutes, they can see the page in much greater clarity because they used their weaker eye.

Repeating this exercise two or three times a day for the first two months, and once a day for the next three months, will forge a whole new pathway in your brain, and the brain will become accustomed to utilizing both eyes in unison.

Accompanied by other exercises that we will do, this will start to wake up the precious macula in both eyes. This is relevant because the macula reflects what is in the universe. One of my workshop participants, a physician by profession, spoke like a poet, and his poetry resonated deeply within me and within the other workshop participants. He said, "The macula is like the sun, and the periphery is like all the stars around the sun, and the farther you get from the sun, the less bright it is. The farther you get from the macula, the dimmer you see. But you would see with dim light."

He was absolutely right. The farther you get from the macula, the less you see bright light and clear details, but the more you see dim light and unlit details. There is a place for both the macula and the periphery. We need to use both. The macula can be stimulated by strong sunlight with the sunning exercise. It is stimulated by your thoughts and by your actions. The more you look at details, smaller details nearby and smaller faraway details, the better you see.

Look far away right now. Look at a cloud. Look into the distance, just like you had learned to do before. As you look far into the distance, you see clouds and mountains, buildings and sky. While you see clouds moving, or mountains on the horizon, wave your hand to the side and look into the distance. Also, pay attention to smaller details than the ones you would normally see. Let's say you see the windows of a faraway building. Now close your eyes and visualize the windows and their frames. Try to recall details within one single window. Then open your eyes and look from window to window. Do not strain to see. Take a look at the absolutely smallest details you can possibly see in one window, as long as you don't strain.

Now close your eyes and visualize a contrast. If you saw a white curtain with a black frame, visualize the differentiation of those colors. If you saw wrinkled curtains, close your eyes and visualize the difference between the wrinkles and the protruding parts; then look up and down that window. From there, start to look at all the rest of the windows. Moving from one to the other will activate your macula. Additionally, you don't lose the periphery and you pay attention to what you see with your weaker eye while waving your hand to the side of the stronger eye.

In most cases, a person's weaker eye for proximity is also his or her weaker eye for distance. However, with a minority of cases—but still a high percentage—it can be that one eye is stronger for seeing near, and the other eye is stronger for distance. If this is the case with you, do this exercise first with your eye that sees well from nearby; then do it with your eye that sees well from far off. This work can make a very big difference to you in that both eyes will participate more equally in whatever you're looking at. As you continue to look from afar, you will see that your eyes get sharper, just like from nearby. As you look at smaller details, the larger ones become clearer because your macula has gained function and can look at a great speed from detail to detail. In fact, the speed is so great that you cannot notice.

You can also examine how well you see from mid-distance. Mid-distance is somewhere between four feet and fifteen feet. You can use the same "fist telescope" technique that was mentioned earlier to tell if one eye is stronger at mid-distance.

Comprehension Problems with the Weaker Eye

A third of those who have disparity between their eyes have comprehension problems with their weaker eye's reading, meaning that they don't necessarily retain what they read with the weaker eye. This exercise works to correct the disparity.

I recommend blocking your strong eye with a small piece of paper taped to the bridge of your nose. Now wave your hand to the side of the strong eye. Read three sentences with your weaker eye; then take the page away and use a tape recorder or MP3 player to record yourself as you repeat, from memory, what you read. Now play the tape back while reading along with the weaker eye; 80 percent of everyone who does this will realize that their retention of information is bad with the weaker eye.

If you have a partner to work with, keep reading the sentences to your partner as you recollect them until you get the sentences right. This will help to build retention with your weaker eye. Before doing this exercise, be sure to palm for six minutes, in addition to sunning and working with both eyes; only then should you isolate the weaker eye.

Step 8: Blocking the Strong Eye

This next exercise, as physical as it is, can also give you a whole new mental outlook of the world. Sunlight is the best lighting in which to do this exercise. Otherwise, very strong interior light will work if it makes it easy for you to see the letters.

Look at the page in front of you from a distance that is comfortable and easy to read. Wave your hand to the side of your head, from all the way above your forehead to the side of your eyes and beneath them. You could also wave around a colored piece of paper, a toy with different colors, a stick with a ribbon, or anything else that draws your attention. Look centrally at the letters on the page while peripherally sensing the object that you wave. As a result you will be working both your periphery and center together. That will release your eye from strain. Your eyes, as I mentioned before, cannot strain if both eyes are being used together.

Whenever there is strain, it is because one eye is being used more than the other. This exercise can make a huge difference by helping you to integrate the center and the periphery. Anytime you are looking at something that you can't easily see, like a menu or a newspaper, wave your hands to the side, and slowly but surely the letters will become clearer to you.

Now take a small piece of paper, approximately one inch by two inches, and tape it to the bridge of your nose so it covers your stronger eye. To make sure you have done this correctly, close your weaker eye and make sure you cannot see the page with the stronger eye that is covered. Then wave to the side of your covered eye and read the page with your weaker eye.

Make no effort when you read with your weaker eye. Any effort that you make will slow down your progress in several ways. It will stop you from adopting the habit of looking with your weaker eye at small areas. If it is strenuous for you to look with your weaker eye, your instincts are going to try to prevent your progress. You only need to make one big effort: the effort to make no effort! This will become easier through relaxation.

You are now waving your hand to the side of your strong eye. Wave quickly. The wrist flips toward your ear, and you make sure that your hand does not move farther than your periphery can see. Your strong eye is truly looking straight at the paper, but the central vision of your strong eye is being put on hold for the moment. The periphery of the stronger eye is being fully used and, in fact, may expand. You will be paying attention to a peripheral view that many people inhibit when they look centrally.

Be sure to relax your face. Your face relaxes when your jaw drops and you have a sense that the cheek is a bit longer. Relax your neck and create a sense that the neck is lengthening a bit. In fact, you can even imagine from time to time that a string lifts your head up and that your neck is lengthening.

Keep waving your hand while reading with your weaker eye. Put the page at a distance where the print can be read with slight effort. Your job is to minimize the effort. The way to do this is to follow each letter as if you are spilling dark ink on it or painting it with a marker, as if you were writing it line by line, point by point. Observe the white of the letter and the black of the letter. When you remove the piece of paper, your two maculae will be working together without one suppressing the other.

Most farsightedness could be reduced and perhaps eliminated with this kind of exercise.

Cheap Sunglasses

Buy yourself some cheap sunglasses and remove the lens from the side of your weak eye. Then cover the other lens with an opaque tape such as dark duct tape. Put the glasses on and look into the distance with your weaker eye.

After you have looked into the distance for a while, take a rubber ball or a tennis ball and play with that ball at a distance. (Have three balls available when you do any exercises requiring a ball so that you will have another on hand when one gets away from you.) For example, you can look at a wall twenty feet away; then take the ball and throw it at the wall ten times and catch it.

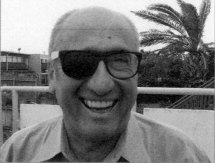

Figure 2.18. The glasses block the central vision of your strong eye while encouraging the peripheral vision to expand.

The ball may not return straight to your hands, but don't lose your patience; just keep playing with it. This exercise helps to develop the lens and also helps with central vision.

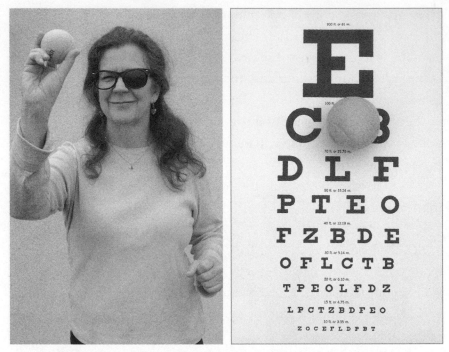

Figure 2.19. (a) Take a ball and throw it so it hits the large letters. (b) Tennis ball hits eye chart.

After doing this for a while, attach an eye chart to a wall. It is best to have two eye charts available: a ten-foot chart and a twenty-foot chart. The twenty-foot chart is especially good for those people whose vision is poor. The ten-foot chart is for those whose eyes are stronger.

Stand five to ten feet away from the charts to look at the first two or three lines. Stand between ten and twenty feet away to see the top six lines; you should not be able to see the bottom four lines too well. Then take a ball and throw it so it hits the large letters of the twenty-foot chart and one of the large letters of the ten-foot chart. Throw the ball and catch it. Do this fifteen times in a row. You may find that you can see an extra line on the eye chart, maybe even two additional lines. Take your glasses off and use both eyes. With both eyes, you most likely will see one to three lines better, and there will be a very nice feeling of clarity of vision through deep relaxation. You allowed the strong eye to rest and the lens of the weak eye to work fully. The lens became flat when the ball hit the chart and round when the ball returned to your hand. And you let your macula work well from afar because the central vision works well when it looks at small details.

Next, you can work with the eye chart the same way in which you worked with the page in front of you. Put the piece of paper on the bridge of your nose to block the central vision of your strong eye. Wave to the side of your strong eye while looking with your weaker eye at the print that you see clearly. For example, if it's easy for you to see the first letter or the first line, but it becomes progressively harder for you to see the second or the third line, then look at the first line, point by point and line by line. Do this as if you were spilling black ink on each of the letters and making them sharper by following the different parts of each letter.

Wave to the side, above, and below your strong eye. Make sure that the strong eye does not see any letter on the chart. (If you close your weaker eye, the paper should block the central vision of your strong eye, and your strong eye would not be able to see the chart.) When you wave your hand to the side of your strong eye and you look with your weaker eye, you wake up the macula and strengthen it. This strengthens the nerve impulses and the muscles of the weaker eye, and it feels good!

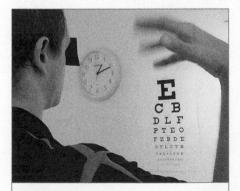

Figure 2.20. Put the piece of paper on the bridge of your nose to block the central vision of your strong eye.

Just as you did with the larger print, look at the smaller print while imagining that you are drawing the shapes of the letters. Many people then see the small print better. Look at the lowest line that you can see (which could be the third, fourth, or fifth line on the chart) as you wave your hand to the side. Now look three lines below and look at the spaces between the letters. If you cannot see the spaces between the letters three lines below, look two lines below; if you cannot see the space between the letters two lines below, look one line below. Always look below your comfort zone at spaces between the print, even though you cannot read the print. Close your eyes and say to yourself, "The ink is black and the page is white," while imagining that your hand is waving on the other side. Saying this makes your brain engage with much smaller spaces from the distance that you can comfortably see the eye chart, whether its five, ten, or twenty feet, depending on your vision.

You will then get engaged with that particular distance, and that engagement gets you to see well from that distance. Keep waving your hand on the side of your strong eye while looking at the print that you cannot really see. After looking from point to point in that print, look back at the line that you could see. Fully half of my workshop participants and private clients can see that line clearer, and some of them could even see an extra line, or a few letters of the extra line, clearer.

One particular optometrist, who attended a workshop of mine, told me this was "eye-opening" for him (no pun intended). And indeed it was. When you take the paper off, you experience that with both eyes you can see a couple of lines below the ones that you saw before, for the two maculae are working together without one suppressing the other. The effort of looking is then diminished, the desire to look increases, and the other exercises that you started to do will work better for you. When you look from a distance, you will make no effort to look at details. They will come and go; slowly and gradually, you will see more and more of them, as far as the horizon and as close as forty yards away.

Look at Details One More Time

As I said earlier, the motivation to look at details is so important. It is nice to see adults wanting to look at something trivial, something that isn't necessary for life, like an animal walking, a beautiful garden, a sunset, or cloud formations. You can't pay your bills with gorgeous skies, but when you look at them in a meaningful way, you're engaging in something significant. When we were kids, we didn't judge anything because we were not capable of earning a living then. We looked at everything out of curiosity—and, indeed, childhood vision is precious and great.

When we lose our curiosity, we lose much of our vision. Through inhibition and the requests of life, we learn to look at letters in order to gain content from them, and sometimes to see a page at a time, without looking at one single dot on that page. We observe other people only in order to understand what their expression means to us for a particular purpose or endeavor. By looking at a food shelf without paying attention to all that's on that shelf, but just looking at the specific item that we need, we soon cut out 90 to 95 percent of the details that the world presents to us. The reason is that we know what we want way too well.

The problem is that we suppress the work of central vision and of the whole eye mechanism. The visual mechanism (the brain) does not pay attention to most details. The eye does the same thing. Many muscles get frozen: the ciliary muscles of the lens get frozen; the iris muscles of the pupils get frozen; and some of the external muscles get frozen as well, since they are not being used. Much of the retina is not working.

I will never forget a time when I saw a father and his daughter looking at some print. She was fifteen and he was in his midforties. She could see print much smaller than he could. He could see down to the fifth-print level, and she could see down to the eighth. I said to him, "At your age, you could see exactly what she sees." After seeing hundreds of kids and how excellent their vision can be compared to the "normal" vision of adults, I could understand that childhood vision, even if it is less than normal, is much better than most adults' vision. The father said to me, "What have I done all my life? I've missed out on something very important." He had done very important things in his life: he was a surgeon, he had operated on people and saved lives, and he read books, but he did not pay attention to his own visual system; day by day, second by second, it decayed. It was clear to him and to me that if he could begin to be vigilant about his visual system and work with it, he could learn to improve his sight. Even after decreasing his visual acuity as much as he had, he was able to gain a lot of acuity that day and saw better.

In the cases of people who have lost retinal cells, renewing an interest and appreciation of details can help them gain back much of their lost vision. Your curiosity and need to look at details increases with these exercises, and you will feel more alive. You will feel that you breathe better and meditate clearer as you go along in life.

Our work, therefore, is to wake ourselves up to look at details and to revive the dormant centers in our brain. Much of the potential we possess is latent and asleep. It's hidden from us because we adopt bad habits that we incorrectly think will work for us.

There is a continuous debate these days about vision. One side believes that simply having normal vision function is sufficient. The other side believes that paying attention to your vision function and working on it constantly is just as important as its functioning. The second group of people is still a minority, but that minority is growing. If you are reading this book and practicing the exercises, you are in the minority that believes we should always work on improving our vision. If you are in the minority, you also believe in vitalizing our vision and giving it life.

These eye exercises and those that follow can help you to see better and to feel better. Make time to do these exercises daily. The most important thing in life is to pay attention to the universe. The universe begins with you and your body. When you pay attention to your eyes, you'll be in better contact with the whole world. You'll also bring more circulation to your eyes, and you'll feel better. Then you can help your own life and will find it is easier for you to help the world.

Sometimes an exercise will work perfectly fine one day, and not the same way the next day. There could be many reasons why this happens. For example, palming will work better if your shoulders are relaxed and worse if they have retained tension. Shifting will work much better if you are refreshed. Blinking (discussed in the next section) will work much better if you have a good night's sleep and if you are relaxed at the time.

One sign that you're doing well is if you find yourself looking at details for no special reason: observing and not ever straining to see them, but always having a sense of all the details in the object you're looking at; you're enjoying the object or looking at it in total neutrality. If you find yourself breathing deeper and absorbing the world with a greater joy, then all these exercises will carry themselves into your day-to-day life and become natural habits.

Step 9: Blink

In order to improve our awareness of blinking, and to receive all the benefits of blinking, we have to have individual control over each eyelid.

One great exercise is simply to open and close each lid separately. Another is to cover one eye with your palm and then concentrate on opening and closing the other eye by itself. Imagine that the eyelashes are doing all the work of opening and closing the eye.

If your eyelids feel dry or sore, you should either palm them or just close your eyes for a while. A reliable way to rest your eyes is to put a hot towel over them and relax them. This will increase the blood flow to your eyes. If you have inflammation in your eyes, putting a cold towel on them will feel nice. Through relaxation, you will discover a profound difference in your ability to blink.

As you look at details, you will find yourself gently blinking. Your eyelids should feel weightless. For a fraction of a second, the eyelids close and then open; it will happen quickly. It will massage your eyeball and trigger moist and pleasant tearing. It will also trigger the widening and contracting of the pupils as you open and close your eyelids. Blinking should be very gentle and pleasant.

When you blink and your eyes feel refreshed, looking at details becomes easy. It sounds counterintuitive to many people, as the feeling is that blinking interferes with looking. Nevertheless, the rest you receive from closing your eyes for a brief moment helps you to move from

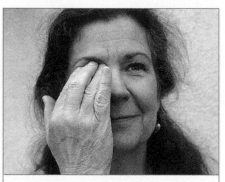

Figure 2.21. Cover the right eyelid with your fingers right underneath the eyebrows, and blink with the other eye.

detail to detail with greater ease. In fact, without that rest, the mind would have a hard time concentrating on any one point. The rest allows you to keep functioning with greater ease. Blinking massages your eyes and brings you more vitality. The desire and willingness to look gives your whole body more life. Relax your forehead. Relax your jaw. Relax your temple. Experience the wonderful sensation of vitality in all of your face and neck and chest and upper body as you blink.

If you sleep well and feel refreshed, if you exercise gently, if you feel relaxed and sense that the blood flows better in your body, you will find yourself blinking with greater ease. And if you blink with greater ease, you will find that you are relaxed and that the blood flows better throughout your whole body. Blinking influences, reflexively, the sense of relaxation and movement in the body. If the jaw drops and doesn't crunch, then the shoulders drop and do not elevate, and the pelvis becomes loose—just from blinking gently, softly, and continuously at a rate of twenty-two to twenty-five blinks per minute. Blinking and looking at fine details is something that most children do automatically. It gives you a sense of youthful energy.

A good blinking exercise is to move your head in a rotating motion in each direction for a total of five minutes, very gently. Performing this motion in medium-sized circles while blinking will bring more blood to the head, which, in turn, will make blinking easier.

Another wonderful exercise is to put one hand underneath the other while gently pressing with your head against your hands and moving your head in a rotating motion in both directions. When you put one hand underneath the other, your hands are steady, and there's the sense that you are bringing much more blood to your face.

A great way to prepare for blinking is to blink in a dark room, where it's easier for the eyes to open and close. Blink three or four hundred times in the dark. Then massage your eyelids very gently. With a very light touch, stretch the eyelid from the eyebrows to the eyelashes several times; then you will start to be ready for one of the most difficult exercises in this book.

To do this exercise, first cover the right eyelid with your fingers right underneath the eyebrows, and blink with the other eye. When you blink, remember to think how the eyelashes are doing the work of blinking. Since your hand is covering your right eye, you can feel how much your eyelid moves when you blink your other eye. The goal here is to be able to blink the uncovered eye without experiencing any movement at all in the covered eye. This is very difficult and requires much practice. You must massage the covered eyelid as well as the forehead while you try to blink only one eye. Massage your forehead and temples gently with your fingertips. Imagine that the eyelashes of the left eye are moving the eyelid and that the forehead is not working, because it is in the muscles in the middle of the forehead where the two eyes merge and unite and one suppresses the other. On a tissue level, you do not want one to suppress the other. Now repeat the exercise while covering your left eye.

If you contract your face in order to blink, then you teach your brain that the muscle that blinks is too weak to do it for itself, and it needs to borrow the forehead muscle. But if you loosen up the forehead and temples and roll the skin of your scalp from the occipital area to the frontal area, you will find that it's easier for your eyelids to be independent. It's so important for us to remind ourselves that light eyelids are eyelids that have healthy circulation. It's amazing how much your sense of well-being improves when your eyelids are light. There is less fatigue all over the body. It is astonishing how tight your face, neck, chest, and upper body are if your eyelids are heavy.

Stroke your eyelids about six or seven times. Then cover one eyelid with your fingers in such a way that the fingertips are under the eyebrows. Do not put your hand on your forehead, because then you will not feel the eyelid. Just underneath the cushions of your fingers you will feel the eyelid, and you will feel how much it moves when you blink.

Blinking will help you to develop your peripheral vision and will remind you not to strain your eyes.

Step 10: Vision and Body

The health of the eyes is intertwined completely with the overall health of the entire body. Blood flow in particular has everything to do with muscular health, cardiovascular health, and relaxation. The following exercises will help you to maintain the health of your entire body while you continue to work on improving your eyes.

Walking Correctly

Walking is a wonderful exercise for staying fit and active. It is a low-impact way of exercising that gets your blood flowing. But it is important to pay attention to how you are walking.

Make sure that you are walking heel to toe, with correct posture: spine straight, chin up, and shoulders back. Do not slouch. Do not let your head droop. Look where you are walking so that your neck is not stiff. Now relax. Do not tense your shoulders; just make sure they are not drooping forward or down. Remember not to strain. Being tense while walking is never good. Relax and enjoy the fresh air and exercise.

It is also good to sometimes walk backward and even sideways.

Rest Your Eyes

We must rest our eyes completely. For 1,500 years, Tibetan Yogis have made it a point to spend extended periods of time sitting in dark caves and meditating on the color black. When they exit the caves, their vision is incredibly good. Just think how much they stretch their pupils!

In the Jewish culture, we meditate on the color blue since we believe, for some reason, that black is the color of sadness, a funeral color. But it isn't sad. In fact, it's a wonderful color, one of total rest for your optic nerve.

Today, because of city lights, we strain by not having fully stretched pupils. When you stretch your muscles, you can then contract them much better also. For example, if you stretch your hamstrings, you will feel much lighter when you walk. The same thing happens to your pupils; it's just that the response is not as quick, so we don't feel it.

The pupil has two round muscles. One muscle widens the pupil, and its collaborator contracts the pupil. To properly stretch both muscles, you need to sun and to night walk; unless your pupil can expand all the way, it will never be able to contract all the way. The more you can constrict your pupil, the clearer your vision will be. Whether your vision is only 20/400 (about 10 percent of normal vision) or 20/40 (85 percent of normal vision), you will end up improving your capacity to see better with constricted pupils.

Quite often, after having a long nighttime walk in an area that doesn't have much light, people who see 20/40 will improve their vision to 20/20. After this, city lights may suddenly start to be a bother. We are learning that city lights disturb the pupils by not allowing them to expand all the way. Of course, city lights aren't completely bad because they can help us find our way. We go to coffee shops as a result of having city lights. We can travel with ease as a result of having city lights. But we never experience the papillary expansion that is so necessary for better vision. The muscle that expands the pupils simply does not work all the way.

After fifty minutes of night walking in the park, the muscle expands all the way, and the whole face and neck relax. The next day, it's much easier to contract these muscles. You will respond much better to the sunning exercise if there is also expansion from looking in the dark.

One way to help your pupils is to do many exercises in a very dark room. To make a room completely dark, close your curtains at night; then play in there with a glow-in-the-dark ball. Relax as you do it. When your eyes open wide in the dark, you will experience relaxation all over your body. Try the Melissa exercise, described in the section "Stretch Your Eye Muscles." Cut a long piece of opaque paper, about two inches wide and the length of your face, and tape it to your forehead and to your chin. Throw the glowing ball from one hand to the other in a tall arc. Throwing the ball can also help your eyes to stretch. You will find that your eyes rotate much easier in the dark.

If your eyelids are fatigued or your eyes hurt, and it is a hot day, lie down and put a cold towel over your eyes for about three or four minutes periodically throughout the day. If it's a cold day, then put a *hot* towel over your eyes. I always found this a great vacation from life. I also found that whenever I worked with patients in San Francisco, where we often have cold air and fog near the ocean, they relaxed themselves and improved their progress if we put hot towels over their faces for awhile. Sometimes, lying down and closing your eyes for four or five minutes can make a very big difference.

Deep relaxation of the eyes, and proper contraction of the pupils in the dark, will lead to more relaxation in normal life and can help us to maintain good vision for life.

The Power of Breath

When you practice blinking, one of the automatic reflexes is slow, deep breathing. The slower your breathing is, the more relaxed you are.

The best way to breathe is slowly in and out through the nose. When you breathe, you want to feel your abdomen expanding when you inhale and shrinking when you exhale. You want to feel your ribs and chest expanding when you breathe in and shrinking when you breathe out. Proper breathing encourages a sense of calmness and relaxation in which blinking and looking at details become easy and natural from moment to moment.

When you breathe, you feel warmth in your hands and feet. You also feel balanced throughout your whole body. When you breathe deeply, light becomes easy for you to absorb.

So let your abdomen and your ribs expand, but also feel your back expanding with each inhalation and shrinking with each exhalation. When we look with ease from detail to detail while blinking with ease, breathing slowly and deeply, and when we become adjusted to strong light, our vision comes alive.

Loosen Your Neck

You can loosen your neck in many different ways. One is simply to look into the distance while you stand erect. Do not let your head

63

move forward. When you're standing erect, there is a ligament that holds your neck straight, just like there is a ligament that holds your lens flat when you look far into a distance. This is a wonderful position for the body.

Since the normal tendency for most people is to bend forward, the neck usually becomes tight. From time to time, stand erect and look far into the distance, and you will maintain a soft neck that will not need any treatment; this will also bring more and more blood flow into your head. Using this technique, you will prevent many problems that relate to poor blood flow to the head.

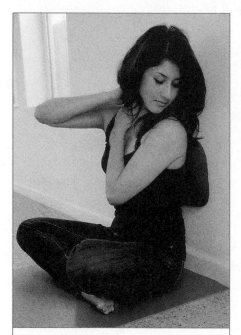

Figure 2.22. Tap with your fingertips on your neck, all the way from the base of your skull to your shoulder, back and forth.

Now, sit in your room on the floor with your back against the wall, with a small pillow that creates an arch in the middle of your back. Put your head against the wall and rotate your head from side to side. As you do this, stretch your neck. Breathe deeply and slowly. Tap with your fingertips on your neck, all the way from the base of your skull to your shoulder, back and forth.

Now, for a brief moment, put your hand on the side of your chin and stretch your neck even farther to the left side; then stretch farther to the right side, while tapping up and down your neck to loosen the muscles. Do not continuously push your head. You will then find that the neck is stretching, and when you move the head from side to side, you'll find that it moves slightly better.

You do not need to do this exercise for more than ten minutes per day. Even so, it will be very valuable in preparing your body for other exercises in this book, because more blood to your head means less pressure in your eyes. And the pressure in your eyes, if abnormal, can cause problems. More blood to your head also means that you have refreshed eyes, and refreshed eyes tend to respond much better to these eye exercises.

More blood to the head has all the benefits I've mentioned and a great many more. It has absolutely no side effects, will make you feel refreshed, and will help you to be alert. It will help you to do what you want, while seeing at ease and seeing well. You will find that moving your eyes from side to side becomes much easier for you when more blood flows to your head, all that can only happen with a loose neck.

Another wonderful relaxation exercise is to lie on your back with your knees bent and your hands to your sides. Now roll from side to side. Your hand will push you to roll to the opposite side. Push with your left hand, and you roll to the right. Push with your right hand, and you roll to the left. Do this about a hundred times every day before meals, for several months, and it will help your neck while increasing the blood flow to your head.

Another wonderful exercise is to sit up, interlace your fingers, stretch your arms out in front of you, and rotate them in a complete circle, in their entire range of motion, whatever that is for you. Visualize that your fingertips are leading the motion. The full movement of the arms loosens up your shoulders. Also, rotate your wrists. The looser your wrists are, the looser your shoulders become.

For the past 150 years, we've had the tendency to not lift our arms all the way. Nowadays, many men and women wear jackets that restrict the movements of their arms. That stiff look of immobile shoulders has been around for too long!

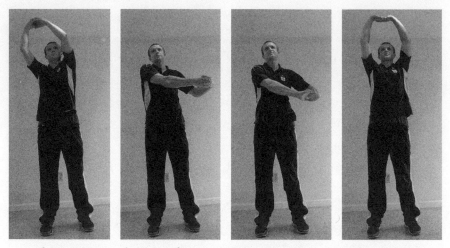

Figure 2.23. Interlace your fingers, stretch your arms out in front of you, and rotate them in a complete circle in both directions.

Our ancestors used to climb trees and lifted their arms upward on a regular basis. We don't, and we're paying a very dear price for it, because not lifting our arms restricts blood flow to the hands, head, and eyes. These days, our fingers are very stiff. We write, we type, we drive, and we constantly contract our fingers. Musicians, sign language interpreters, and massage therapists like me tend to contract their fingers even more. We don't balance this movement with enough extension. Many workplace injuries and arthritic conditions happen because of stiffness in the wrist and fingers.

Interlace your fingers and point your palms outward while moving your arms in a rotating motion in both directions. This

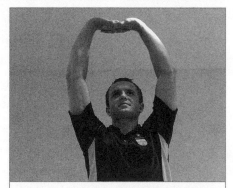

Figure 2.24. Now point your palms outward while moving your shoulders in a rotating motion in both directions. Circle your arms up.

position helps you to stretch your hands and prevents lots of other problems. If you feel a nice stretch in your forearm, you have done your job. I remember a woman who took my class and had such poor circulation in her hands that they looked green. When she practiced stretching her hands and wrists, and moving her shoulders in a rotating motion, however, they became pink.

Stretch Your Eye Muscles

Here's a wonderful way to stretch your external eye muscles and relax your neck: tape a long strip of nose-width paper from your forehead to your chin and throw a ball from hand to hand, back and forth.

A student of mine named Melissa was in a terrible accident in which a pick-up truck ran over her body and head and broke many of her skull bones. Consequently, she was subjected to more than twenty surgeries on her face. One of the surgeries was on her deep orbit, and the recovery from it was very difficult. She developed extreme double vision and neck pain. When we put the small, medium, and large pieces of paper between her eyes, she saw well peripherally but saw double below and above those papers; her neck kept hurting as well. When we placed the big piece of paper from her forehead to her chin and she threw the balls from hand to hand, her neck stopped hurting, at first temporarily, then long-term.

This practice of putting a long piece of paper from forehead to chin has become known as the Melissa exercise. You simply tape a piece of paper to your forehead, then tape the bottom of the paper to your chin, and do exercises while wearing this paper. It may not immediately feel as much of a neck relief to you as it did to Melissa, because your eyes may not see double and you may not experience that extreme difference. Nevertheless, it may feel like a great relief for you from the strain of one eye that controls the other; this relief immediately leads to better vision for more than 60 percent of the people who do this exercise.

With the paper on your face, throw a ball from hand to hand for five to ten minutes. You will see the ball in your right hand with your right eye, and when the ball crosses in front of your face, you will see it with your left eye as you catch it with your left hand. Only one eye can see the ball at one time. Throw the ball from hand to hand, allowing each eye to work separately as you try to catch the ball. If you have access to a trampoline, it is wonderful to do this exercise on it while you bounce.

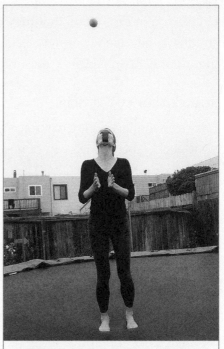

Figure 2.25. The Melissa exercise.

Many other variations of the Melissa exercise are covered elsewhere in this book, but this is the basic starting point: throwing a ball from hand to hand while the paper is taped to your forehead and chin.

You may find that this eye-hand coordination, with a clear divider between your two eyes, can make a big difference and can help you to relax your eyes. Keep doing the shifting exercise, which will also stimulate the macula. When you are refreshed, the macula works better, and all other parts of the eye work better as well.

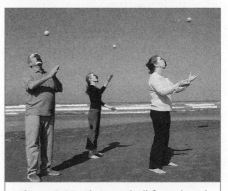

Figure 2.26. Throw a ball from hand to hand while the paper is taped from your forehead to your chin.

Enjoy the View

Often, pleasant scenery appears in front of us—faraway places with beautiful views. But even people on vacation are entrenched in the habit of not looking. They will only spend a few minutes, here and there, actually looking at the view. Then they will go on to deal with their vacation plans and work-related issues involving computers. A reason for this is that they are not used to looking at the beauty that attracts one's vision on a daily basis.

Some people do not have anything beautiful to look at in their workplace. Nor do they have anything beautiful to look at in their residence. But most people in the world do have access to beautiful places to look at, somewhere in their lives: a nice garden, beautiful plants, lovely pictures, and even changing clouds.

Develop the daily habit of looking at something pleasant. We should devote twenty minutes a day, divided into four-minute increments, to looking at something beautiful. It could be combined with the looking into the distance exercise, or it could be apart from it. Spend a few minutes every single day looking at beautiful scenery, and it will slowly instill in you the desire to look at details. Then, when you go for a vacation, instead of spending twenty minutes looking at nice details in nature, you may end up spending two or three hours doing just that, and still enjoying yourself.

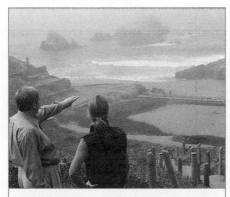

Figure 2.27. Looking at the distance relaxes the eyes if you don't strain to see.

We are creatures of habit. Whatever we do now will perpetuate what we will do later. Create new habits of looking at details: first with your lenses, then without your lenses, then with reduced lenses, then again without your lenses, then maybe with pinhole glasses (discussed in the next chapter) that help the pupillary contraction, and finally without lenses or glasses again. If we enjoy looking at details, we will develop a skill that is lost by modern life, and that skill is the ultimate fortress of strength for our visual systems.

If you have vibrant, healthy, and mobile eyes, as you look at objects, you will also relax your whole body, which will feel vibrant and thus looser and more mobile. Because the eyes lead the body, the body's posture arranges itself around the way the eyes see. Therefore, making your eyes more alive can trigger your whole body to come alive.

If you focus on your breathing and visualize expansion and contraction, you mimic the movement of the whole universe, which is in constant motion, expanding and shrinking. When you begin to sense this, and move in that direction, it can give you a pleasurable relaxing sensation that you may never have had before. If you combine the visualization of blackness with the expansion and contraction of your body, you start to have a sense of an inner rhythm that you never had before.

Repetition of these exercises gives you a pleasant sense of relaxation that augments your sleep, but the benefits go much deeper. When your conscious brain learns to relax, not only will it relax when you palm, it will relax *anytime* you look. And that is exactly what you want to do: consciously relax so that your subconscious will start to work in a whole new way.

Don't Squint

Your tendency to squint is one of the highest hurdles on the path to vision improvement. Squinting is a manifestation of physical and mental resistance toward improvement and change. If you do not squint your eyes much in the light, your brain demands that the pupils contract; when they do, your vision becomes much clearer. If you do not squint when you read, you will start to look with a soft eye at the print on the page.

Ready to Move On

I would like to congratulate you if you have earnestly worked on yourself using all the principles and exercises we've discussed so far, because it means you are devoted to your health and to your life. And who is going to help you if not yourself?

There is an old Jewish proverb: if not now, when? If I am not going to take care of myself, then who will? It is an illusion to think that others can do better for you than you yourself. So continue to practice with my suggestions, and you will feel the difference. Your vision will improve, and you will maintain your vision for life.

Chapter 3

Computer Use and Relieving Built-Up Fatigue

When working at a computer terminal, it's critical to be aware of your position, the lighting, and your overall surroundings. First of all, you should sit at a distance from which you can comfortably read the screen. There should be adequate lighting (natural light is best), but it should not be shining directly into your eyes; nor should it be reflecting off the screen, creating a glare. Finally, the computer itself should be positioned where you can easily gaze into the distance: next to a window or a long hallway would be a good location.

You can use the features of a computer to your benefit by following data as it appears on the screen or by visually keeping track of the movement of your fingers across the keyboard. Look at the actual shapes of the letters you are typing and be aware of the spaces between them.

Often, however, when we work at computers, we create an "invisible strain" that we don't really feel. This is the worst kind because if you don't recognize the strain, you will do nothing about it. And if you are actually straining, then by the end of a day of computer use, your eyes may be red and you will be unnecessarily fatigued.

So, what is it that actually makes you strain as you look at a computer screen? First is the weariness of looking from so close. If you look into the distance three times a day for eight minutes, it can help to alleviate this. Not everyone, however, has this amount of time, so even twice a day would suffice. This can occur before you start to work, after two hours of working, or at the end of the work day (if your eyes are not too tired). The main thing is not to strain: do not try to *see* the distance; instead, *scan* the distance. From time to time, use the obstructive lenses described in Step 8 to obstruct the eye that sees better from far away, even if the other eye sees better from near. Then take the glasses off and keep looking into the distance.

Every hour that you use a computer, you should do something different. If you focus on the rush of information coming from your monitor for very long, it's very easy to disregard your peripheral vision. When this happens, your central vision becomes overtaxed, a situation that may contribute to glaucoma or lead to a loss of clear vision. So it's imperative to provide your central cells with some rest by stimulating your peripheral cells. You can accomplish this by doing the peripheral vision exercises, which will enable you to notice the periphery more: you acknowledge the floor, the wall, the ceiling, and your general work environment. When the periphery is being used, you won't tense your eyes as much.

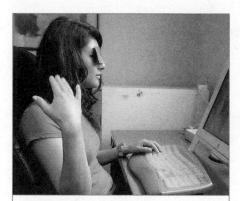

Figure 3.1. It's imperative to provide your central cells with some rest by stimulating your peripheral cells.

The long swing can also work wonders because it gets you away from your computer terminal and forces you to do something physical with your entire body along with your eyes. Even if you have only a few minutes to do this, there will be a noticeable improvement in your vision when you return to your computer. The Melissa exercise is also wonderful to do every day for five minutes; place it anywhere in your day when your eyes are not so tired that they won't respond to an exercise. In this way, fatigue does not accumulate. Palming for a minimum of six minutes could also be beneficial at some point in your workday, preferably after not more than an hour of sitting at your computer. If you make palming an intrinsic part of your daily routine, it will help your eyes to recover from any strain they are undergoing. And, as your day progresses, you should alternate between all of the aforementioned exercises in order to obtain the most beneficial results.

Throughout your entire workday, you should be certain to pay attention to the periphery as well as the fact that your two eyes are looking. From time to time, as you are reading the computer screen, put a small piece of paper in front of your nose, covering the strong eye. Then wave your hand to the side of the strong eye and read with your weaker eye. Close your eyes and try to remember the last line you read, and say it to yourself twice. This helps because sometimes the brain will remember only what you read with the stronger eye, and this will force you to read with both eyes.

While working, it's a good practice to look away from the computer for fifteen seconds every half hour. When your day is entirely over, it's good to finish up with a ritual of three minutes of peripheral vision exercises and one minute of doing the long swing. By doing this, the drawbacks of computer work will not affect you as much; in fact, you may even be encouraged to exercise your eyes more.

There are basically two problems that result from using a computer. One is that we are just not meant to stare at a computer for eight hours a day. Our ancestors did not do it, and through them we have developed the kind of eyes that we currently possess. Nowadays, however, nearsightedness is increasing at an astounding rate. When Dr. Bates was devastated about schoolchildren in New York in the 1920s, it was because 6 percent of them were nearsighted. These days, we would like to return to what had already been thought of as a large percentage, because 48 percent of kids who attend school in the United States today are nearsighted. Sadly, the numbers are even higher in other places around the world: in Hong Kong, it is 62 percent; in Taiwan, it is 84 percent. Therefore, the entire world needs to start to understand these implications. And while the computer itself may not account for these results, looking from near for lengths of time at a stretch *is* partially responsible for them. This mode of working tempts you not to use your periphery, which is what triggers the problem in the first place.

The other difficulty is that pixels have unique properties, and it's harder for the eye to see them even though we don't sense it at the time. The cumulative effect over a period of hours of computer use, however, is substantial. Hence the importance of taking our eyes away from the screen periodically. It is also essential to blink frequently yet gently as we are working. Not only will this break you away from the fixation of staring at your computer screen, which contributes to eyestrain, but it will serve to moisten your eyes and to reduce tension in the muscles around them. Burning, inflamed, or itchy eyes will eventually be alleviated by blinking.

From time to time, especially when you feel you are not responsive to any of the exercises, just massage around the eye orbits, from the bridge of the nose to the temples and from the nose to the ears. Relax yourself, even if it means only ten strokes (about twenty seconds) of this, which could really remove the fatigue you have accumulated. Now, if you're working on a hot day, you could end up having invisible inflammation in your eyes. So lie down once a day with a cold, damp towel around your eyes.

You need to campaign for zero tolerance in building up unnoticed fatigue. First, you need to be aware of its existence; then you need to remove your fatigue as you progress through your day.

The detrimental thing about reading from a computer screen is that we have incorrectly learned to read only the document in front of us, and not to pay attention to our eyes. If we have bloodshot eyes, we go to an ophthalmologist and get eye drops, thinking that fatigue does not affect the eyes adversely. But once it begins to accumulate, nothing will go right with your vision. And this could be prevented by managing that fatigue. It's very important to take a day off sometimes. During that day, don't use a computer; instead, do some eye exercises. It is also beneficial to take time off during each day and not look at a computer screen; designate times for using your computer and times when you won't be using it. Naturally, this will vary with the individual, and whereas some people prefer to enjoy their day, using their computers only at nighttime, others will prefer just the opposite. Once you have decided on the hours you will not be working, you can revive yourself from use of the computer by doing other things and by paying more attention to everything it kept you from using, like your peripheral vision or your weaker eye. Otherwise, by looking from near you can strain one eye; looking from far, you can strain the other.

In conclusion, value your eyes as much as you value the material with which you are working. Similarly, value your breath just as much as you value your project. The moment you make these decisions, the computer will never harm your eyes. If your decision is to ignore them, however, the computer can harm your eyes big time. And never believe people who tell you that a computer can't damage your eyes, for their advice alone can damage you as well.

Chapter 4

Improving and Correcting Errors of Refraction

In this chapter you will find specific exercise programs I recommend for the treatment and, at times, the reversal of vision problems related to errors of refraction. These include myopia, hyperopia, presbyopia, and astigmatism. Although this chapter specifically focuses on errors of refraction, the exercises discussed here will aid in the treatment of many conditions discussed in Chapters 5 and 6. These include cross-sightedness, cataracts, diabetes, glaucoma, optic neuritis, detached retinas, vitreous detachment, macular degeneration, and retinitis pigmentosa.

If you are currently under the care of a physician who is open to a holistic approach to healing, I encourage you to share this information with him. Together you will be able to monitor your progress and adapt my suggestions to your particular condition. These exercises are intended to work in conjunction with whatever else you are doing to heal and maintain your vision.

As I mentioned in the preface of this book, many doctors are quick to prescribe chemicals and even surgery to correct all problems including vision problems, and they will often discourage you from believing that your condition can ever return to normal, regardless of whatever efforts you might be willing to make.

What, after all, is the definition of healing? Healing does not always mean an instantaneous cure, a total reversal of every ailment.

Sometimes that happens, but more often, true healing comes in small steps. True healing is simply an improvement, however minor, within the parameters of what is possible given the circumstances of your life. It is important to make comparisons only with yourself. If you can improve, however slightly, from where you are today, give yourself the validation of acknowledging that small success. Build upon it and celebrate it. Celebrate every small accomplishment along the way, and remember where you started.

I cannot stress enough how much faith I have in people's ability to heal themselves through the diligent practice of these programs. My personal experience of working with myself, with my children, and with thousands of patients and students has taught me that improvement is possible and that the benefits of these exercises are tangible and well within your reach.

Suggestions for Using This Part of the Book

First, make sure you have familiarized yourself with the basic exercises explained in the earlier sections of this book. I will refer back to them again and again. Now turn to the section in this chapter that addresses your particular vision condition. Follow the exercises I recommend for at least the time periods I suggest in each section. Most important, make a commitment to incorporate these exercises into every aspect of your daily routine. I may recommend six minutes of palming or ten minutes of sunning, but this is only a starting point: the bare minimum. Ideally, instead of setting aside one part of your day to do these exercises, you will find moments throughout your day to exercise so that the improvement of your vision is always at the forefront of your mind. Don't stop being conscious of your eyes and the ways in which they function throughout the day. Never stop looking at details.

Think of this part of the book as a starting point. As with muscular exercise, the best program is not simply to work out thirty minutes a day, three times a week, while being sedentary the rest of the time. The best idea is to incorporate movement and physical exercise into every aspect of your life. Walk throughout the day. Take the stairs instead of the elevator. Do push-ups and sit-ups whenever you have a few minutes to spare. Stretch. This way, you are always exercising and always aware of your physical condition.

The same principle is important here. Start with my recommended time periods for these exercises, but learn to always find time throughout your day to palm, to sun, and to look at details. Accordingly, awareness of your vision will become ubiquitous and will be a priority to you no matter what else you are engaged in throughout the days and weeks of your normal life.

Make a long-term commitment to the program and take time out to measure your progress regularly. Do not give up. Do not set unrealistic expectations of instantaneous healing. Take every success, no matter how small, and build upon it. Keep a journal of your progress and your feelings along the way.

If, at any point, you feel as though the exercises are taking you in the wrong direction or are not creating the benefits you desire, it is possible you could benefit from additional therapy. There are classes all the time at my School for Self-Healing in San Francisco (www.self-healing.org), and I also offer off-campus lectures and therapy sessions around the world. I encourage you to research possible opportunities to work with me or with one of my trained practitioners if you believe it could benefit you in your quest for better vision.

Where Do Corrective Lenses Fit into These Exercises?

Ideally, as long as it doesn't cause you stress or strain, you will practice improving your vision without wearing your lenses, at least part of the time. Once you are a month into doing your exercises, go to a friendly optometrist that does not oppose your working on your eyes, and ask for a pair of glasses that corrects them to 20/40, which is 80 percent of 20/20. When your eyes see better with those new lenses, go back and get a new pair with an even lower prescription. Getting used to the lower prescriptions will build your eyesight.

Some people with very severe myopia (nearsightedness), of 20/500 or lesser vision, should have three different pairs of lenses: 20/20 glasses to drive with safely on foggy nights; 20/40 glasses to walk around with in the daytime; and 20/80 glasses with which to challenge themselves while walking around in a familiar environment. In most cases, after two months of this, you will be able to see 20/20 through the 20/40 glasses. Then you can return to the optometrist and change back to the 20/40 prescription once again, which will be the *new* 20/40. The idea is to reduce the strength of your current eyeglasses in increments until no glasses are needed at all. We expect you to reduce two diopters a year and to see better all the time. Of course, the rate of progress will vary from person to person.

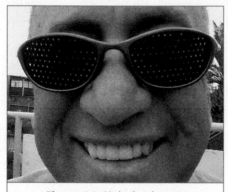

Figure 4.1. Pinhole glasses.

At a certain point, when you feel comfortable walking outdoors without glasses, we suggest you get a pair of pinhole glasses and put them in your pocket. Look at people's faces and signs up close without glasses. When you are at a distance at which the signs or faces are not as clear, however, put on the pinhole glasses and use them to read signs or recognize faces.

Also, you can use the pinhole glasses while reading. First, look far into the distance for a few minutes to rest your eyes; just look without trying to see anything in particular. Then read without glasses for fifteen or twenty minutes and look into the distance again. Next, read with pinholes for a half hour and look into the distance again. Finally, read with your regular prescription. This exercise is not perfect for everyone, but it can be adjusted to fit your situation. What should never be compromised is that you should never strain your eyes to read.

Pay attention to your individual abilities; if you can hold on longer with the pinholes, that is fine. What you want is simple: to gradually transition out of the continuous use of your glasses.

If your myopia is not severe (i.e., if you see 20/200 or better), my suggestion is to walk everywhere without glasses, unless you drive or have a specific safety reason that requires you to wear glasses. Meanwhile, keep the pinhole glasses in your pocket. When you see a sign that you can read, but with difficulties, or that you can hardly read but can follow some of the shapes, put on the pinhole glasses and look at the sign again. Often, the pinhole glasses will help a person see the sign better. Pinhole glasses work with two-thirds of people, but not with everyone. Pinhole glasses also work with most of my students, but they do not work with me. They either work for you, or they don't. Since they are not expensive, however, it is worth your while to try them and find out.

Correcting Myopia and Hyperopia

Imagine that you are using a projector to show a film. If you have placed the screen too far away from the projector, farther than the focal point of the lens, the image will be blurry. To someone with myopia, this is how the world looks. Things nearby are clear, but things far-away are fuzzy. With hyperopia, it is as if the screen has been placed too close to the projector. Things close by are fuzzy, but things farther away are clear. With presbyopia, the lens is too stiff, so nothing can be clear from nearby because light is not being allowed in correctly.

Myopia

Myopia is a vision disorder in which a person can clearly see nearby objects while objects in the distance appear blurry. Also called near-sightedness, myopia occurs when the eyeball has become too elongated, and light entering the eye isn't focused correctly; this is what causes distant objects to appear blurry.

High myopia is an extreme case of nearsightedness requiring more than eight diopters of correction, and it progresses consistently. Though you see well with correction, the eyeball continues to become longer and longer, which causes the retina to become thin, thus risking detachment. This detachment deprives the photoreceptors of vital nutrients and can lead to blindness. There are many other severe problems besides retinal detachment, such as glaucoma and macular degeneration, which can occur if your vision does not improve without glasses. As your vision improves, the eyeball regains its normal round shape.

We can see how one problem leads to another if we don't take care all the time to improve our eyes.

Beneficial exercises for correcting myopia include shifting, palming, peripheral exercises, reading with pinhole glasses, and night walking. Devote at least one hour a day to these exercises, and remember not to pack the entire hour into just one part of the day. Find time throughout the day to work on your vision. Try a session of night walking once a week. If you live in an environment where it is not safe to night walk, you may wish to substitute walking around and moving in a dark room for forty-five minutes; this can wake up the rods through movement, although there is really no perfect substitute for walking outdoors at night.

Once you begin to experience improvement, you may want to increase the recommended time periods for each exercise. This is a good idea and can lead to even more improvement in your vision. In truth, my recommended hour of exercise should be considered a minimum starting point. If you have very severe myopia, you may want to start with an hour a day, and as you experience improvement, you can move up to two hours a day or more. An hour one day might seem extensive if you are busy, but on another day it may not be a big deal to spend several hours!

Exercise Program for Myopia

- Night Walking: 45 minutes, once a week.
- Shifting: 10 minutes daily for the first two months; 5 minutes daily after that, and throughout the day, with 30 seconds here and 30 seconds there. You should find minutes here and there to pay attention to details until it becomes subconscious. From time to time, you can check on yourself and see that you are constantly looking from detail to detail, all the time progressing to smaller ones.
- Palming: 20 minutes daily.
- Peripheral Exercises: 10 minutes daily.
- Bouncing the Ball: an extra exercise for myopia.

For this last exercise you will need a tennis ball, an eye chart, and your sunglasses, with its lenses popped out and the strong eye's lens obstructed with opaque tape. You should have your eye chart posted on the wall at eye level. Basically, what you are going to do is put the glasses on and throw the tennis ball at a line on the eye chart and try to catch the ball again. But it is a little more complicated than that.

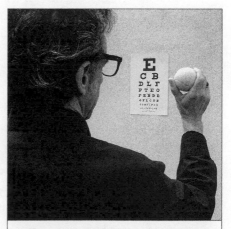

Figure 4.2. Wear your obstruction glasses covering the strong eye and throw the ball at the chart.

Stand in front of the eye chart at a distance from which you can read the top three lines well, the middle lines with more difficulty, and the bottom lines as being completely fuzzy. This is the correct distance from which you have the opportunity to make improvement. You should not be closer than three feet away, but whatever distance beyond three feet that is comfortable for you should be okay. It is important not to judge yourself harshly about what distance is comfortable for you. If five feet is your distance, work to achieve improvement at five feet; if seven feet is your comfortable distance, work to achieve improvement at seven feet. Remember that you are seeking something very personal and should only compare yourself to yourself.

So, put on your cheap sunglasses, the ones with the strong eye's side blocked with opaque tape. Pick up the tennis ball and extend your hand out toward the eye chart. Aim the ball at one of the largest letters on the chart. Retract and extend your arm several times, as though you were taking careful aim. Visualize that the ball is hitting the chart and flying back into your hand. Now throw the ball at the chart and try to catch it again.

Repeat this exercise from all the different angles you can. Throw the ball at an angle from one side; throw it at an angle from the other side. Throw it overhand and underhand. Throw it with a lob; then throw it straight out in front of you. Now take the glasses off and look at the chart again.

Let's assume that when you started, you saw the first three lines quite well but, from there down, it started to get fuzzy. After throwing the ball, look at the eighth line and focus on the spaces between the print. Then look back at the sixth line and see if the letters have become clearer. Focus on one letter on the sixth line and then close your eyes and say, "The ink is black and the page is white." Say it five times, open your eyes, and look at the print again.

Now put on the glasses again and throw the ball back at the eye chart. Repeating this exercise often yields positive temporary results and, over time, gradually improves many people's ability to see lower lines on the chart.

A variation can be done while running in place. For this variation, attach a medium strip of black paper to the bridge of your nose so it obstructs your strong eye. Now run in place and bounce the ball on the eye chart, catching it again if you can. Wave your other hand in the periphery of your strong eye. You wave your hand to the side of the stronger eye so it can only pay attention to the periphery, provided that you are looking straight at the paper that obstructs it. Your job is to never lose track of the hand that is being waved to the side. The important thing here is to get your two eyes working together. The reason that you run in place is to keep yourself moving, so you will not freeze your gaze. Breaking the tendency to freeze is the beginning of better vision.

The next step is to run in place with the paper obstructing your strong eye and to throw the ball back and forth with another person. Do not put the paper in the middle of your eyes. Make sure you are obstructing the strong eye so that you are working on both the periphery of the strong eye and the central vision of the weaker eye.

When you look at the eye chart before beginning this exercise, look at the lowest visible line, where you can see most of the letters but not all of them. Pick a letter you can see clearly. Close your eyes, visualize the letter, and say it out loud. For example, if it is a Z that you can see clearly, say, "The Z looks clear. The Z looks wonderful. The Z is black and the page is white." This is just to appreciate what you see. Enjoy the fact that you see the letter clearly. Instead of saying, "I don't see clearly," you are saying, "This is what I do see, and it is wonderful." This is positive reinforcement, but you are doing it in a very tangible way. The Z *is* wonderful! Even if it looks fuzzy, you enjoy the way it looks anyway. Respect what you have and work with it.

I have met quite a few people who compare their vision without glasses to their vision with glasses, and they are not enjoying the vision they have. Allowing yourself to enjoy the vision you have, however, is where the healing begins. It's like the old adage that the one who is rich is the one who is happy with his fair share. You're talking about a field in which people are so emotional and so aware of what isn't there, without ever really being grateful with what they can actually produce. Say, "The O is great! The A is great!"

Now look back at the chart and see if you can identify more letters. If you can, be grateful because the very fact that you can breaks the concept that many doctors are stuck in—that the eyes cannot improve—which is bogus! The improvement may be temporary, but it will show you the possibility that daily repetition of this exercise will help your myopia to improve over time.

While practicing this exercise, you must experience definite improvement from the distance that you have designated for yourself before you change your distance. Some people are tempted to change their distance too quickly. For example, they see really well from five feet, after not seeing well from five feet, so they move quickly to ten feet. Nevertheless, you have to understand that the eye of a nearsighted person is very rigid, and the mind of a nearsighted person is fixated with the vision he or she has.

So, if you improve from five feet, enjoy your improvement. Get used to the clarity from that distance. Experience and love it. Enjoy the fact that you see better and that you can measure your improvement. Stay at that distance for six months before you increase the distance by two feet. When you experience improvement from your new distance, stay there for six months; then increase three more feet. The gradual improvement is the permanent one. It needs daily work, and you can't neglect it.

One additional exercise is to look at the eye chart from a distance that is comfortable for you. Look at a line that you can almost read; then move up two lines from there to letters that you can easily read but that are not sharp. Now take a sheet of paper and make an entire page of letters that size. Create for yourself two pages of random letters, with anywhere from twelve to twenty letters on the page. If your vision is highly challenged, use as many sheets of paper together to give yourself at least twelve different letters to look at. Now hang your paper next to the chart, read it from the exact same distance you read the chart before, and allow your eyes to become comfortable focusing at that distance. To ensure that you are truly focusing on that letter size, read them from left to right and right to left, up, down, and diagonally, so that you don't simply recite the letters. This exercise is best done with direct sunlight on the page. You can also do this same exercise wearing the cheap sunglasses and looking with only the weaker eye. Reestablish the letter size that is comfortable, but not sharp, with the weaker eye. Repeat the steps above; then return to your original page with both eyes.

You have to keep working until the results are satisfactory. Sometimes you may take a break from exercises, or sometimes you will change them. Instead of always doing one program, you can deviate to keep your mind fresh and to keep engaged in your exercises; this way you will not get bored. Then, you will go back to the original exercises. Be patient with yourself because all vision improvement has to do with inner patience.

An Additional Note about Myopia

Most people with myopia have a good focal point somewhere. Let's say someone sees well from a foot away. That person should do the eye exercises involving eye charts and pictures, and anything that can help with looking at details and shifting, from a distance of thirteen inches, then from fourteen inches. One inch at a time will make it possible to develop vision from afar. Inch yourself ahead of where you are. And remember to do it in strong light like sunlight, or indoors with a light of 200 watts or more. You will find that the light improves your capacity to see smaller details from a slightly farther distance.

That's all you want to achieve: to see slightly better and better all the time. Again, daily work is key. You might change the exercises or focus on different areas, but you must keep working.

Hyperopia

Hyperopia is a condition in which you have a short eyeball. With hyperopia, because the eyeball is short, a picture coming into the eye falls behind the retina. So when it hits the retina, it does not appear clearly.

Since the eyeball is short, you may see fuzzy from nearby or from far away, and you may not have a good focal point from either distance.

The normal prescription for myopia is reduction (minus) lenses. Hyperopia, before being cured by natural vision improvement exercises, is corrected with plus lenses (magnification). Plus lenses are also used by children who were born with cataracts, because they had their natural lenses surgically removed. All can be helped with natural vision improvement exercises.

Many children before the age of six have hyperopia, where they see well from afar but not so well from nearby. So it is very important to remember that when you teach your child to read before the age of six, you may cause eyestrain. Before this age, it is better for children to look at pictures and shapes than it is to look at letters. If you do teach your child how to read early, use large print.

Conventional wisdom says that it is normal for people to grow farsighted when they hit their midforties. In fact, people don't even call it an eye problem. Instead, they say it's a part of the aging process. This is an amazing misconception, and one that I personally cannot accept. Are arthritis or type II and III diabetes part of the aging process? Truthfully, if you develop the correct habits, you can live to the end of your life without developing any of these disorders.

And there is also a way to prevent farsightedness. Be very flexible with your neck and your head and practice the following exercise program every day. Remember: do not simply set aside one part of the day to work on your eyes. Find time throughout your day to work on your eyes so these exercises can become a part of your lifestyle, a constant memory through which you are always consciously working on your vision.

Exercise Program for Hyperopia:
90 Minutes a Day

- Sunning: 10 minutes daily.
- Peripheral Exercises: Pay attention to the periphery all the time, and do at least 20 minutes of intensive peripheral exercises each day.
- Palming: 12 minutes daily.
- Look Far into the Distance: 20 minutes daily.
- Extreme Close-Up: 20 minutes daily.

Prior to doing this last exercise, make sure you look far into the distance; then palm for at least six minutes. Because you have hyperopia, looking at nearby objects is undesirable for you, and you have become accustomed to looking at objects from afar. So now you should train yourself to do the exact opposite.

Find an object that is pleasant to look at, like a flower or a painting. Stand a foot away from your chosen object. Now put your face about two or three inches away from the object and wave your hands to the sides of your face while looking at different details. Then go back to standing a foot away and determine if you can see the object any better. If you find that you can, it means that you have temporarily relaxed the lens muscles and that your lens has temporarily become more flexible and less rigid. In terms of presbyopia, it also means that you may have elongated the eyeball temporarily.

Next, move your eyes in a rotating motion. Look up, look to one side, look down, and look to the other side. Now put your thumb

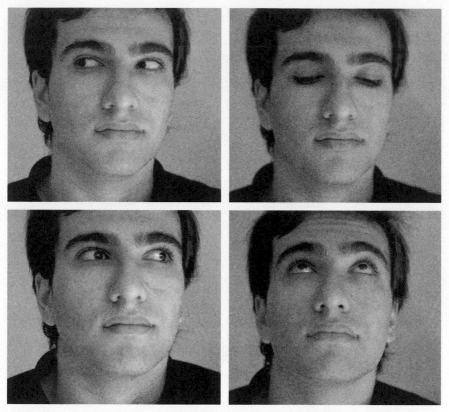

Figure 4.3. Move your eyes in a rotating motion.

and your index finger on the bridge of your nose. Move them up and down while looking at your nails. Look at the two nails from two sides as you look up and down. As you look at the nails, you will find that you are straining quite a bit. Most (meaning 99.9 percent) people cannot see the two nails at once. So, you start with your two fingers above the bridge of your nose at an area where the bridge of your nose meets your forehead. You then move them one centimeter below your nose, and you keep going up and down, up and down, trying to watch the nails. After two minutes of this, look back at the nearby object from one foot away, and see whether it appears clearer to you now. Now look far into the distance for two minutes; then look back at the object in front of you again. Your eyes should have relaxed significantly.

Be aware that you are exercising. This is not a normal way to use your eyes. This exercise is also great for presbyopia.

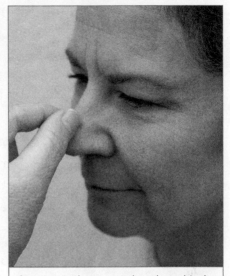

Figure 4.4. Place your thumb and index finger on the bridge of your nose and watch your nails as you slide your fingers up and down your nose.

Correcting Presbyopia

Warning: We have to understand that with hyperopia and presbyopia there could also be astigmatism. So before you do these exercises, it is good to first do the astigmatism exercises. Especially good is the exercise in which you wave the page with large print in front of your eyes while looking at the eye chart. This really takes away the astigmatism.

Hyperopia and presbyopia are similar conditions. The difference is that presbyopia is a stiffening of the lens that occurs through use of the eyes, usually when someone is around forty years old. This condition makes it difficult to focus on nearby objects. Often, people who develop presbyopia start to wear reading glasses to help them focus on books and newspapers or other objects at close range. Hyperopia, on the other hand, is a short eyeball, a condition you are either born with or that occurs because of a modification of the eyes.

The prevailing concept among most doctors is that once your lens is stiff, it can never become flexible again. This is the only reason why people don't work for more flexibility: they have been incorrectly told that it is impossible!

If you are able to arrest that concept and understand that your lens is all-powerful and capable of responding to these exercises, you will never be presbyotic again. Furthermore, you will maintain good reading vision into your midnineties or early hundreds.

Exercise Program for Presbyopia: 60–90 Minutes a Day

(Work mostly outdoors at first. As you improve, work in gradually dimmer and dimmer light. And remember: don't squint!)

- Extreme Close-Up: 20 minutes daily.
- Peripheral Exercises (using the opaque piece of paper between the eyes): 10 minutes daily.
- Bouncing the Ball: 5 minutes daily.
- Look Far into the Distance: 20 minutes daily, divided into two or three sessions.
- Rotate the Eyes: 5 minutes daily.
- Massage around the Eyes: 10 minutes daily.
- Extra Exercises for Presbyopia: 10 minutes daily.

It is important to reiterate the necessity to work on these exercises throughout your day. Even though I suggest 10 minutes of a particular exercise, it is better to do a few minutes here and a few minutes there to get into the habit of constantly working on improving your eyesight.

Extra Exercises for Presbyopia

Blinking One Eye

In this exercise, you are going to practice blinking with each eye separately.

As I have mentioned before, when you close one eye at a time, your brain learns to allow the two eyes to function independently. The way to do this is to close one eye as if you were blinking with it and then to cover it with your hand. Now take your hand off your eye and open it. Repeat this a hundred times for each eye. Afterward, you will find that you have a bit more control with each eye. Although you do this as a concentrated exercise, remember to blink gently throughout the whole day.

Reading in Dim Light

First, practice reading in dimmer and dimmer light each time you read. Now have someone turn the lights on and off while you are trying to read. Next, practice some of your other exercises, like reading large and small print or bouncing a ball in dim light as well.

This practice will improve your vision in strong light within four months. It will also improve your vision in normal light within ten months and will help you to see in dim light within sixteen months. No longer will you be dependent on glasses, which will be a great thing for you.

Look Near/Look Far

For this exercise you will want to find something that it is very pleasant for you to look at, like a beautiful picture. Look very closely at the object. Now put a small piece of black paper on the bridge of your nose so it obstructs your strong eye. Then look closely at the picture while waving your hand in the periphery of your strong eye. Next, look away from the picture and far into the distance. Continue to wave your hand in the periphery of your strong eye. Now look back at the picture again, this time close-up. Take the paper off your nose and look back into the distance with both eyes. Now look back at the picture close in front of you with both eyes. You may be able to notice more details this time. Palm for six minutes in order to relax your eyes. Remember to stop and relax anytime you are feeling strained. The object is not to strain but to relax your eyes, your neck, and your body.

Headlines and Large and Small Print

For some of the exercises that follow, these pages with text of gradually decreasing size will be helpful.

-1-

What is computer vision syndrome? It is, according to the

-2-

American Opto-metric Associa-tion, "the complex of eye and vision problems

-3-

related to near work which are experienced during or related to computer use." The AOA developed this diagnosis after seeing an

-4-

increase in the number of patients requiring eye exams due to symptoms they experienced at the computer. The visual stress of working at computers can bring on nearsightedness (myopia) or make it worse, and can also worsen middle-aged farsightedness (presbyopia).

-5-

CVS is a repetitive strain injury. One muscle that is strained is the ciliary muscle, a muscle within the eye that changes the shape of the lens to determine the focus. Pixels, which make up the images we see on the computer screen, are bright in the middle and blurry on the edges;

-6-

the brain is unable to determine a focal length for pixels, and endlessly attempts to do so. The iris, a muscle within the eye that regulates the amount of light that enters the eye, is strained by inappropriate lighting and glare, which are often a problem with computer work, and the result is light sensitivity.

1
LARGE AND SMALL PRINT

Nothing is more surprising than change, when it arrives—but nothing is more predictable. When we get into our forties, most of us begin to have trouble reading small print. The newspaper becomes easier to read if we hold it out at arm's length.

2
LARGE AND SMALL PRINT

People who have always had 20/20 vision start to walk around with reading glasses in shirt pockets or hanging from a cord around their necks, and those who are nearsighted switch to bifocals. Doctors assure us that it's a common change at middle age; our ciliary muscles, which change the shape of the lens to focus the eye for near vision, weaken, and the lenses become stiffer as we age. What they don't tell us is that the lenses can get even worse—eventually we can get cataracts, the biggest cause of blindness throughout the world.

3
LARGE AND SMALL PRINT

It's not a lack of compassion that causes eye doctors to go on prescribing ever-thicker glasses without warning us of the dangers that lie ahead. They simply feel that it's hopeless, that our eyes can only get worse. Schneider and other vision improvement teachers believe that eyes can also get better. They say that ophthalmologists are seeing only one end of a continuous spectrum—whether you see nothing more than lights and shadows or have vision that is more acute than 20/20, you're somewhere on the continuum, and change in either direction is possible.

4
LARGE AND SMALL PRINT

Even when your eyes are working hardest, trying to make out small print in dim light, for example, they need to function out of a sense of relaxation; this is the bottom line. This is why upper body massage is so important for good eye care.

The eye's own built-in massage, blinking, gets curtailed with the frozen stare that is the hallmark of bad vision.

Blinking bathes and refreshes the eye, gives it intermittent rest, and promotes flexible use—for example, if you're blinking while walking, your eyes open each time to slightly different scenes.

Unbalanced vision/movement patterns create tension in the eyes and poor vision; thus, massage therapists can help clients improve their eyesight by working with them on posture. Midback, shoulder, and head posture are especially important—if the head is habitually tilted forward, for example, the brain assumes that distance vision is limited, and it does indeed get worse.

5
LARGE AND SMALL PRINT

The eye exercises teach relaxed use:

To adjust the eye through relaxation to all intensities of light;

To balance the use of both eyes together. Uneven use creates enormous tension; the domination of the stronger eye needs to be limited, and the weaker eye needs to be strengthened. If one eye, or part of one eye, is damaged—even to the point where it can do no more than register the presence of light—it should be stimulated; the stronger eye will relax, and its vision will improve when the brain senses greater balance;

To balance central with peripheral vision. By habitually gazing at books or computer screens for hours at a stretch, we tend to ignore peripheral visual information until the periphery actually shrinks;

To create a flexible, fluid eye so that the eyes move easily between near and far;

To stop freezing the gaze and shift the eye easily from one small detail to another, lightly skimming the world like a butterfly.

6
LARGE AND SMALL PRINT

You may feel that wearing glasses relaxes your eyes; some people say they feel undressed and unready to meet the world without them. They do create problems—they teach us that without their help, we can only see poorly. They also tend to make us lose peripheral vision, since we are used to limiting our reality to what is visible within their frames.

7
LARGE AND SMALL PRINT

Of all the eye exercises, palming—a visualization of blackness coupled with awareness of soft, expansive deep breathing—is the most important. A meditation in its own right, it can relax the eyes, quiet the senses, and bring calm to an overwrought nervous system. Palming can be done passively to clients, or you can massage their necks and shoulders while they palm. It is a powerful tool. Long palming sessions can be harmful with glaucoma. Massage is a good substitute. Combined with breathing and movement exercises, massage can create a deep awareness of upper-body tension, especially around the eyes, so that the client learns to release it.

8
LARGE AND SMALL PRINT

The "cone" cells of the retina supply daytime color vision in sharply realized detail. To supply central vision, the normally sighted eye is continuously moving, easily and accurately, from one small, clear detail to another—the behavior called shifting. The periphery is supplied by "rod" cells. Although our vision is incredibly high-resolution—we have 100 to 200 million rods and cones—we don't all see all the parts of the visual field equally well. With normal vision, we see one small detail best, in a field of increasing haziness. Accepting this can be hard for near-sighted people, who often find blurriness unpleasant. Because the brain fills in what we expect to see, the entire periphery appears to have color, but it doesn't. Try standing in an unfamiliar room with many small colored objects, looking straight ahead; you wont be able to identify the colors at the edges of your visual field.

Creating Controlled Stress on the Ciliary Muscle for Strength

Ideally, this exercise should be done outdoors on a bright day, with sunlight falling directly on the page. The next best method would be in bright daylight without direct sun. And the least ideal way would be indoors with strong light, which should still work.

Look at the pages with large and small print. Read the normal size print at a normal distance, where the letters are clear but not crisp, and not completely comfortable to read. You might not be able to make out a letter or two, or perhaps even a word or two, but you should be able to read most of it. Do not strain; just look at the letters. Make sure to blink and wave one hand around your periphery to ensure that you don't strain. This will also help you to see well because it encourages the brain to notice more of the periphery and not to overstrain your central vision.

Next, obstruct your strong eye with a small piece of black paper (two inches by two inches) and look at the largest print. Bring the page all the way to your face until the page is almost touching your eyelashes, even closer than the tip of your nose. Read the print, letter by letter, or part of each letter, point by point, reading aloud and waving your hand in the periphery of the obstructed strong eye. Instead of moving your eyes the way you would when you normally read, you will move the paper so that each letter falls right in front of your

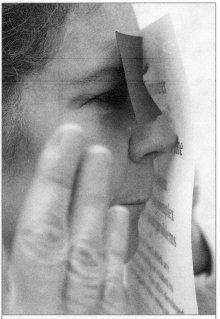

Figure 4.5. Bring the page all the way to your face until the page is almost touching your eyelashes.

eye, in your focal point. Wave your hand in the periphery to take the strain off reading so close. Do this for two minutes.

Now hold the paper back eighteen inches and read the normal print again. This is an induced stress on the eye rather than one of which we are unaware and that strains the eye. Nevertheless, this will strengthen the ciliary muscle. In 80 percent of my clients and students, this works both momentarily and, with continued practice, long-term.

Unfreezing

It is amazing how much our patterns control us. If you tend not to move much because you watch television a lot, sit at a computer all day, or drive for a living, it can eventually lead to a frozen back, a frozen gaze, frozen looks, and, quite often, repetitive thoughts in your brain. Even if you are intellectually very advanced, you may freeze the way in which you look and the way in which you move.

If you are a long-distance runner, you may run with a constant sense of freeze, meaning that you tighten your shoulders, neck, chest, and lower back when you run. Or if you lift weights, you may tense every part of your body in order to lift them. So, a sense of freeze may be the starting point from which you function.

One of the most important things for you to learn is how to unfreeze yourself. Regardless of what your lifestyle is, you could be frozen.

If your lifestyle is one of sitting, it's important for you to be comfortable when you sit, not just to *think* that you're comfortable. You should be properly supported in your seat so that you do not damage your back and neck from freezing your posture. It's likewise important to know that your eyes are relaxed, not frozen. How do you know that your eyes are relaxed? Simple: first of all, they blink; second, you have a sense of periphery when you look straight ahead.

Eye exercises are the beginning of unfreezing. Body movement is also the beginning of unfreezing. Unfreezing is more than a thing to do—it is a philosophy that you share.

Correcting Astigmatism

Astigmatism is caused by an irregularly shaped cornea or an irregularly shaped lens. It is difficult to describe what the world looks like to people who experience astigmatism. Oftentimes, people with astigmatism have the sense that they see several images of objects at once. For example, when they look at the moon they may see the image of a clear moon along with a shadow moon, two shadow moons, or several shadow moons side by side. Even if they close one eye, they may still see more than one moon.

Often astigmatism accompanies nearsightedness or farsightedness. Thus a progressive way of improving your eyes would be to simultaneously work on correcting the myopia or hyperopia while also addressing the astigmatism.

After practicing the recommended exercise program for astigmatism for two months, the astigmatism may disappear. It is then advisable to return to these exercises for one week every six months, for several years, in order to prevent the astigmatism from recurring.

Note for Astigmatic Readers

Beyond your program, you must do extra looking into the distance and extra palming throughout your day. Even though you do the astigmatism program, when you sit at your computer again for four hours or so, the benefit you have gained with these exercises is going to decrease. By regularly looking into the distance and palming, you give your eyes the opportunity to rest and to maintain more of the progress you have made with your vision.

Therefore, you must take moments throughout your day to add to your program. If you have been looking closely at your computer screen for an hour, take some time and look into the distance. Palm two or three times a day, for no less than six minutes each time, but don't forget to blink and to breathe freely and deeply.

Exercise Program for Astigmatism

- Sunning: 10 minutes daily.
- Palming: 12 minutes minimum, 6 minutes at a time.
- Headlines: 20 minutes daily.
- Glow in the Dark: 20 minutes daily.

Extra Exercises for Astigmatism

Headlines

Note: If you are farsighted, this is a great exercise to practice before starting to work on your other exercises.

For this exercise, you will need an eye chart taped to the wall at eye level, your cheap sunglasses with the lens on the strong eye's side

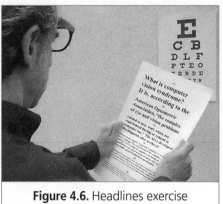

Figure 4.6. Headlines exercise for astigmatism.

covered with opaque tape, and the page with large and small print or a newspaper with a large-print headline.

Stand at a distance from the eye chart so that you can see the top third of the chart clearly without much straining, but you have to strain to see the bottom two-thirds. Basically, you are going to look at the eye chart while quickly waving the headlines in front of your face. Look past the blur of the headlines being waved in your face and try to read the eye chart. Every few seconds, stop waving the headlines and look quickly at them. Blurt out the first letter you see clearly. Now wave the page back and forth again and go back to reading the eye chart. The object is to quickly shift your focus from far to near and back to far again.

If you have a partner with whom to practice these exercises, you can do this exercise a little differently. While you are reading the eye chart, your partner can flash fingers in front of your face, very close to your eyes, and you can tell your partner how many fingers he or she is holding up. Of course, this method is not good if you are by yourself because you cannot surprise yourself with your own fingers!

So when you are practicing by yourself, pick up the page with the large headline and quickly wave it back and forth in front of your eyes while looking at the chart. Read the chart aloud even if all you can read is

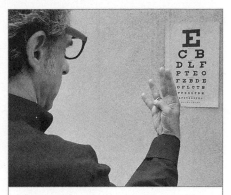

Figure 4.7. Variation on the headlines exercise for astigmatism.

the first three lines; do so repeatedly. Now for less than half a second, stop waving the headlines, look at the large print, and say the first letter you can see. If you are in a phase of half-guessing and half-seeing because of the speed, that's exactly where you want you to be. Then return to waving the page back and forth.

Let's say that you are reading the letters on the top line of the eye chart. As you wave the piece of paper with the headline back and forth in front of your face, you might see the words "moving economy" in your periphery. What you want to do is to wave the paper so quickly that when you stop you may only see "e"; then you keep waving it and say the letter "e" as you return your gaze to the chart and read the top line of letters once again. Then you stop waving the paper, and you may see the letter "c" or the letter "o." Announce it aloud; then wave the paper and read the top line of the chart again. It is good to speak with a loud voice as you do these eye exercises, as it helps to distract yourself from focusing on the exercise itself. This will make it much more effective.

The next phase is to improve your near vision by trying this same exercise reading the large and small print on pages 99–100. This way, you are working with the eye chart to improve your eyesight for distant objects and with the large and small print pages for objects nearby.

Now put on your cheap sunglasses with the strong eye's side covered with opaque tape. Again wave the paper with the large print in front of your weaker eye while looking at the chart. Read the top line of the chart aloud while waving the headline back and forth in front of your face. From time to time, stop waving the headlines in front of your face for half a second, enough time to guess a letter that you see. After ten times of doing this, look at the chart with your weak eye, but without waving the headline in the air. You may be able to clearly read an extra line on the chart. Then take off the glasses, and you may be able to clearly read two extra lines on the chart.

Glow in the Dark

Note: We do this exercise because we want the eye to move around. We have found, in our experience, that many people have an easier time moving their eyes in a rotating motion in the dark.

The idea is to follow the glowing objects with your eye, not by moving your whole head. Move your eyes only, so that your eye muscles are stretching. The stretching motion changes the structure of the eyes with time. People say the cornea cannot change shape, but they are wrong.

For this exercise, you will need a glow-in-the-dark ball, a dark room, and a strip of paper to tape to your nose. The paper should stretch from the top of your forehead to the bottom of your chin, the same as in the Melissa exercise mentioned earlier in this book and also in the next chapter.

Eventually this exercise gets simple, but it's difficult to master at first. All you do is tape the paper to your forehead and to your chin, turn the lights off in your room, and play catch with the glowing ball. Throw the ball from hand to hand so that the ball crosses the visual plane in front of your face. It should disappear briefly as it passes the paper taped to your head. You can also practice bouncing the ball off the wall, throwing it with one hand and catching it with the other. Remember not to move your whole head to track the location of the ball. Move only your eyeballs so that they can stretch through their full range of motion in both directions.

Imagine doing curls with your biceps but only bending your arms a little bit. You would not be getting the full benefit of the exercise, and you may even damage the very part of your body you are attempting to build up. This idea is the same when it comes to your eyes. Exercise the eye muscles by watching the glowing ball in the dark and moving your eyes through the full range of their possible motion; this will stretch, and even change, the shape of your cornea over time.

Chapter 5

Overcoming Cross-Sightedness and Lazy Eye

Correcting Cross-Sightedness

Amblyopia and strabismus are both terms for cross-sightedness, and they have something in common. They both refer to a "lazy eye," but with amblyopia the eyes do not look cross-sighted from the outside. With strabismus, however, the eyes actually look crossed.

I have heard people sometimes joke that strabismus is when one eye is so beautiful that the other eye just wants to look at it all the time! It is okay to have a sense of humor. And this really is true: every part of you is beautiful, even your strabismus!

With amblyopia and strabismus, the brain shuts off the information coming from one eye, but only in strabismus do the eyes look crossed to the outside observer. And the term "lazy eye" is actually a misnomer. In reality, the brain is just not using one of the eyes.

If you have cross-sightedness, you have two problems. One is that your brain favors one eye over the other. This causes one of your eyes to do all the work while the other eye relaxes, which is why some people refer to cross-sighted people as having a "lazy eye."

The other problem with strabismus, or amblyopia, is that doctors do not believe you can improve your condition in any way. Doctors mistakenly believe that, after the age of eight, cross-sighted people can no longer learn how to get their two eyes to work together.

The debate over the plasticity or elasticity of the brain is ongoing, but old concepts are giving way to new understandings. More and more people understand that the brain can change if it's being exercised properly.

As I mentioned earlier in this book, the oldest person I've worked with so far was 101 years old. He experienced great changes from his exercises, and he was able to see better and to improve his brain and eye function significantly. I have also worked with several elderly patients, some in their eighties and nineties, and have witnessed positive changes in their visual systems. There is no doubt in my mind that no matter what age you are, you can change the function of your eyes; there is enough elasticity in your brain to back it up.

The issue isn't age, but whether or not a person is practicing the correct exercises for his or her age. It may work easier for a five-year-old child to put on a patch for four or eight hours a day as he or she plays in order to get used to the weaker eye working. Indeed, the brain has more plasticity when you're five than when you're seventy-five. But, there are good, age-appropriate exercises you can do at any age that can change your visual system completely.

In addition to the exercises in this section, it is essential to do some of the previously mentioned exercises as well. Especially helpful for cross-sightedness is the exercise in the section on astigmatism called "Glow in the Dark." As I mentioned in the introduction to Chapter 4, it is important to refer back to that chapter for an extensive explanation of the exercises I recommend in this section. In addition to extensively describing the exercise steps, there is important information regarding the benefits of these recommended practices.

One other wonderful practice for you is to lie down twice a day with a warm towel over your closed eyes. One of the recommendations that I normally make is to soak the towel in warm herbal tea. Do not use boiling water, just warm water. Within two or three minutes, the towel tends to cool off, and that pleasant feeling can improve your circulation and increase your level of relaxation when you start to work for further improvement. The reason to do this with the towels is to alleviate the strain you have caused your eyes after doing the other exercises. Relaxation must be something you prioritize after doing all of them. Alleviate the strain with a wet towel!

Also, and this is especially vital for cross-sightedness, make sure you are practicing breathing exercises daily and receiving face, neck, and back massages from a certified massage therapist at least once a month, but preferably much more often.

Exercise Program for Cross-Sightedness: At Least 90 Minutes a Day

- Sunning: 10 minutes daily.
- Palming: 12 minutes daily.
- Long Swing: 10 minutes daily.
- Glow in the Dark: 10 minutes daily.
- Walking Backward: 5 minutes daily.
- Blink Each Eye Independently: 5 minutes daily.
- Extra Exercise for Cross-Sightedness: 30 minutes daily.

I cannot stress enough how important it is to make these exercises a regular part of your daily routine. Whatever you are doing, you can also practice your eye exercises. While you are waiting for a bus, you can do your sunning. While you are riding the bus, you can look far into the distance. You can always be looking at details. At work, instead of taking cigarette or coffee breaks, take breaks to practice long swinging or palming. Anywhere there is a dark room, you can practice throwing a glow-in-the-dark ball around! Don't just practice for one hour or two hours at home. Incorporate these exercises into every aspect of your life. That is the way to give yourself good vision for life!

For your extra daily exercise, you may choose from any of the following. The main point with cross-sightedness is to train the brain to use both eyes, not to favor one eye over the other. All of the following extra exercises do just that.

Extra Exercises for Cross-Sightedness

Rotate the Eyes; Look into the Darkness

Sit in a dark room, looking straight ahead. Sit up and don't lie down for this exercise. Now move your eyes in a rotating motion in the dark. Within a few minutes, even a dark room seems to have some light. Move your eyes from area to area in the dark room. Look up, and move the eyes from side to side in the room; then look down, and move your eyes from side to side while the eyes are looking down. Now close one eye and slowly move the full range of rotation with the open eye: up, to the side, and down. Then switch which eye is closed, and repeat. We do this to stretch the external muscles, which, to some extent, are responsible for the cross-sightedness.

Mirror Images

The next exercise uses a mirror. If your left eye is the one that turns in, look in the mirror while covering the right eye. Normally, when you cover the right eye, the left eye should be totally straight because the two retinas and the two eyes are not competing; but sometimes it isn't. In this case, tilt your head a bit to the right and look intensively at the left side, and let the right eye be straighter. Do this several times and palm for thirty seconds to relax your eyes.

Now look at the bridge of your nose. Do not look at the right eye; do not look at the left eye. Look at the bridge of your nose between both eyes, and you will see both eyes. If they tend to cross, this is exactly what your brain will correct automatically. For your brain, normally, is not as aware of the cross-sightedness as you may think. You may see it in pictures. You may even sense it from time to time. But when you face the mirror and look in between your eyes, so your central vision is on the bridge of your nose and your peripheral vision is from both sides, you can exactly see the cross-sightedness. It's amazing how much the brain tends to correct what appears to be wrong, and the cross-sightedness can decrease. If the eye tends to tremor a bit, the tremor will stop.

In addition to this exercise, as you stand in front of the mirror, move your hips in a rotating motion. Don't stop looking in the mirror while your hips are moving. The movement helps to distract you, but it also helps you to get more circulation to your eyes. If the hips are loose, the ribs will be looser, and your breathing will get deeper. Your neck will get loose as well, and more blood will flow to your eyes.

Quite often, the shortening of one muscle, versus the lengthening of its opponent, has to do with poor blood flow to that muscle. So remember to move your hips in a rotating motion when you look in the mirror. If your vision is good, you can do this in any light. In fact, dim light may be the best light you can do it in, because it rests the eyes. If your vision is poor, you may need a strong light to see your face in the mirror.

By now you know that anytime there is an indication of effort in doing this exercise or any other, you must palm. Palming will help you to reduce the stress and to renew the work. Also, you can look into the distance before doing the mirror exercise.

I found that my mirror exercise was one of the best exercises to reduce my strabismus. You see, I struggled with strabismus from a very young age. In fact, in my case, the eyes never communicated because I was blind around the time that most people have their eyes working together, which is between four and six months of age. Since I was blind during that time, my brain had never developed straight eyes. In 1992, at the age of 38, I received my passport picture, and my eyes were severely cross-sighted. Six months before the expiration of that passport, the Brazilian Consulate issued me a five-year visa stamped on that passport. New pictures were taken in 2002, when I was 48, so I had two passports to compare. I took these passports to my school. Before going to the Brazilian Consulate to verify that I could use both passports, my good colleague and student looked at the passport pictures and said, "My goodness, look how your eyes have improved!" My cross-sightedness had decreased, and my eyes had straightened by 75 percent in ten years. Since then, I laugh at the fact that I lost hair and grew older by ten years, and yet my eyes got straighter. Now, years later, my eyes are even straighter. And so, straightening your eyes is definitely possible between your forties and fifties, but it is also possible in your seventies and eighties. You just need to do the work.

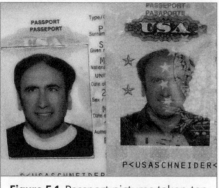

Figure 5.1. Passport pictures taken ten years apart. My eyes had straightened by 75 percent.

Looking in a mirror was one of my main exercises. I used to stand in elevators if they had good light and, for a moment, look in a mirror at the bridge of my nose between both eyes. Often, however, people with cross-sightedness look far into a distance, and their cross-sightedness is decreased; sometimes it disappears. The reason is deep relaxation of the eyes.

The Melissa Exercise

The most wonderful exercise for cross-sightedness is the Melissa exercise. As mentioned earlier, Melissa, who works with me these days, had an accident in which her face, chest, and ribs were crushed by a truck. She had a great many reconstructive surgeries on her face. After one of these surgeries, her eye turned in and lost a lot of vision. She also saw double. The exercise of putting a small piece of paper in the middle of the face, then using a large piece of paper and waving to the side, was useful, but she saw double below and above it. So I simply devised a piece of paper that I would place on her nose so that it stretched from her forehead to her chin. I put masking tape on the top and bottom and had her throw a ball from hand to hand. She could see the ball with each eye, and her vision was not double for a while; this provided great relief for her visual system as well as her neck, for her neck hurt constantly due to the unevenness of her eyes.

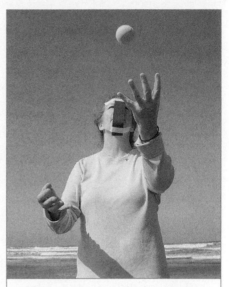

This is a great exercise to help people with cross-sightedness. If you put a piece of paper between your eyes and throw a ball from side to side, at least a hundred times for about two minutes, the ball will disappear for a split second before you see the ball again

Figure 5.2. As you do this exercise (the Melissa), the brain will use both eyes independently.

with the other eye. That will create a very nice difference in your eyes. The dominant eye will no longer control the eye that trails.

To a great extent, that's the essence of all amblyopia and strabismus: a lazy eye. And a lazy eye is not lazy on its own. Often, it's an eye that doesn't see well. Sometimes, however, it's an eye that sees very well, but the brain is not using it. The brain did not learn to use both eyes together, and so, throughout your life, one eye looked and the other one trailed. Until now, the brain did not learn to use both eyes together; it used only the strong or dominant eye. As you do this exercise, the brain will use both eyes independently.

With this division between the two eyes, each eye looks and sees the ball independently. The right eye will see the ball in the right hand;

the left eye will see the ball in the left hand. There is a body/eye connection here that makes it very real for the body and the eyes. This is not a peripheral exercise. In fact, look at the ball. When you throw the ball from the right to the left or the left to the right, there is a moment when you do not see the ball as you throw it above your head. That's good because in a short moment you will see the ball, and your hand will have to respond to what you see. Eye/hand coordination is very precious in this case because it makes it real to your brain that you are actually using the lazy eye, as well as the eye you always use. It's not our purpose to use the lazy eye more than the eye that is always used. Our purpose in this exercise is to use both of them.

The use of both eyes may give you great relief. If it is hard for you to do a hundred repetitions, then start with ten, and palm after taking the paper off. If it's easy, continue to do it three or four times a day. And, if that's easy, then do it for ten minutes three times a day for a month. You will feel much looser, and your muscles will work much better. This happens for two reasons: first, because each eye works independently, which is a big, important first step; second, because each eye looks down and up to follow the ball.

The Melissa Exercise is very important for cross-sightedness, and I recommend that you practice it often. Try the following variations:

Clap: Throw the ball from hand to hand while wearing the piece of paper, and clap your hands before you catch the ball. That will really distract you and will also activate you in a way that will have your brain building new pathways to be able to see with the weaker eye.

So, for example, if your left eye is your weaker eye and you clap your hands before you catch the ball with one hand, it's going to be easier for you to catch the ball on the right side than on the left side. With enough practice, however, it's going to be easy to catch on both sides, and it's going to start to be natural for you to see with your weaker eye.

Walk: Next is to walk as you throw the ball from hand to hand. Walk forward while throwing the ball from hand to hand. Walk backward. Walk sideways. It should become more and more challenging but also more and more relaxing for your eyes.

Jump: Now try to jump when you throw the ball from hand to hand. Jump on the ground or, if you are able to, on a trampoline, which is the best method. You will see the periphery moving in the background while wearing the Melissa paper on your face. You'll also be throwing the ball from hand to hand and trying to catch it each time you bounce.

Combinations: Challenge yourself to combine all levels of the Melissa exercise. Walk while throwing the ball from hand to hand, and also clap your hands before you catch the ball. Walk backward and sideways while you combine clapping. Combine clapping with jumping or bouncing on the trampoline. Or, finally, the most difficult variation of the Melissa exercise is to keep both eyes open, throw the ball up, and then close the eye that does not need to see the ball.

For example, with your two eyes open, throw the ball from the right hand to the left hand. As the ball reaches the area above your head, close your right eye, and with the left eye you will see the ball. Catch the ball with your left hand and then open both eyes. Throw the ball above your head again and, as the ball reaches the area above your head where the two eyes cannot see, close your left eye and catch the ball with your right hand.

Do this for a while and then go back to the original Melissa exercise. Perform the most basic variation, keeping your two eyes open, while throwing the ball above your head and catching it. See how much you have improved, and how simple this original method seems now that you have expanded your comfort zone and have adapted to your new challenges.

Beads on a String

Your job in this exercise is to teach your brain what to focus on and what not to focus on.

First, make a string of beads with five different colors of beads on it. (We have many of these available for purchase at the School for Self-Healing.) Tie one end of the string of beads to something in front of you, like the back of a chair or the railing of your patio. Now hold the string of beads in front of your eyes. Focus on the different colored beads. As you focus on each separate bead, every bead that you focus on must appear to be a single bead. Every bead that you don't focus on must appear to be doubled.

For example, if you have five beads, when you focus on the first bead, the second, third, fourth, and fifth beads should appear to be doubled. When you focus on the third, the first two and last two should look doubled, and the middle should look single. When you focus on the fifth bead, the first four should look doubled, and the last one should look single.

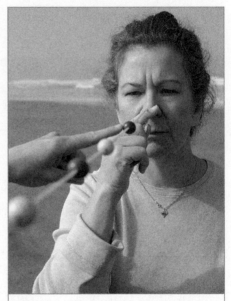

Figure 5.3. Your job in this exercise is to teach your brain what to focus on and what not to focus on.

What often happens to people with cross-sightedness is that, first of all, they may not see double with the beads that are in their periphery; they may see single beads all along. The best exercise to correct this is to look at one bead, let's say the closest one to you, and close your eyes one at a time. When you close your eyes one at a time, you can see a shift, a move of the beads from side to side. While doing this, keep thinking and focusing on the bead in front of you, with each eye separately. That means you keep looking at that bead, but you will see all the beads shifting because each eye sees the bead from a different angle, and even from a different distance. Only when both eyes are open can your brain measure the distances more precisely. After doing it forty times, open both eyes, and when you look at the first bead, the rest should appear to be doubled.

The bead you are focusing on is being viewed with your central vision. The ones you are not directly looking at are being viewed with your peripheral vision. The nervous system and the brain see one image with central vision and two separate images with peripheral vision. When you look at an object straight in front of you but focus on another object in front of *that* object, the object you focus on will appear to be single, and the one you don't focus on will appear to be doubled. You want to become capable of distinguishing between the one you look at directly and the one that you don't, so that the one you are looking at appears to be single and the one you aren't looking at appears to be doubled.

Holding Double

If you were able to see double, the next point is to hold the double. You will find that most people who can produce a double image can hold it for thirty seconds, maybe even a whole minute, before they become fatigued. When this happens, of course, they should massage around their eyes, palm or sun, look into the distance, or do long swinging until the fatigue goes away. You can blink as you do the exercise, and, hopefully, you won't lose the double image.

Your goal is to be able to hold a double for a full ten minutes. You can move from one double to another. You can see the front bead as single and all the other four as doubles. You can move through the five beads, one after another, and hold each double for two minutes. So, you don't have to stay at one point for the full ten minutes, but you should continuously see double for the duration.

You can then increase the amount of time that you see double, and try to go all the way to twenty minutes, or even to half an hour. You can decide one time, in a marathon session, to look at one bead and see the other four as doubles for ten minutes each; therefore, you would see double for fifty minutes. As long as the strain is not too high, this is a great exercise for good coordination between the two eyes.

Two-Color Exercise (Beak Glasses)

This exercise uses a tool we sometimes refer to in fun as "beak glasses." We call them beak glasses because they are glass frames with the lenses removed and with two strips of paper attached to the

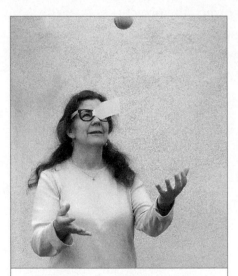

Figure 5.4. "Beak Glasses." When the ball is on the right side, it emphasizes to the right eye that the right color exists.

front of them in such a way that they stick straight out between the lenses. When you put them on, it looks as if you had a two-colored beak.

The pieces of paper should be two different colors; for example, one could be orange and the other yellow. Put on the glasses and look straight ahead into the distance. Now toss a tennis ball from one hand to the other and try to catch the ball. Toss the ball several times.

Since the paper is attached to the front of the glasses, you are guaranteed to be using both of your eyes for this exercise. When the ball is on the left side of your body, it emphasizes to the left eye that the left color exists. When the ball is on the right side, it emphasizes to the right eye that the right color exists. As the ball travels from side to side, the peripheral vision of both eyes is being worked individually; the central vision is still looking straight ahead into the distance. Remember that the central vision sees a mostly still picture, while the peripheral vision sees movement.

One interesting thing about this exercise is to notice which color each eye seems to be seeing. If your eyes are completely at ease and completely functional, when you look into the distance you will see the two colors, each one of them on the opposite side. And this will indicate that they work well together.

If one of these colors disappears, you can also wave your hand close to your eye—not so close that it's dangerous, but right in front of the eye. Often, that color will reappear. Seeing two colors with both eyes, especially for someone who has a hard time using both eyes together, could be a very relaxing experience at certain times.

Red and Green Glasses

Each color has different wavelengths. For example, the color red has long wavelengths, and the color green has short wavelengths. If you look through a pair of glasses with one green lens and one red lens, quite often the colors of the objects you look at seem to be different through the red lens than through the green. Some colors you can see easier with the red, and others you can see easier with the green.

When you look at the world with both eyes through the red and green filter, you will see quite

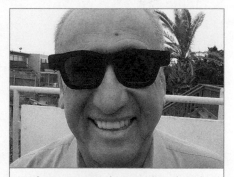

Figure 5.5. Working with red and green glasses made it possible for me to have partial three-dimensional vision.

a few amazing things. For example, if you walk in a park or in your garden with red and green glasses on, you're going to find that you see a pinkish view of flowers through the red lens but, at the same time, a greenish view of leaves much clearer with your green lens. So, from time to time, close one eye and look at colors with the open eye; then close that eye and open the other, and see what colors you notice. Do the pink flower petals disappear when you close the eye looking through the red lens? Do the green leaves disappear when you look only through the red lens? Now look around with both eyes open.

You'll find, however, that if you close the eye looking through the red lens and look at the pink or reddish flower only through the green lens, it will not look red or pink to you; rather, it will look dark, which is far from its true color. If you close the eye looking through the green lens and look only through the red, the green leaves would look dark.

In fact, this is exactly how you start to develop bilateral vision and three-dimensional vision. You emphasize to yourself the difference between the two eyes. Your two eyes are independent. No one eye sees what the other one sees; therefore, no one eye controls the other. Instead, each is independent of the other, and the brain fuses the image from both of them equally.

In the past, I had no three-dimensional vision. I didn't know if an object was close to me or far away from me. But as I improved my clarity, I wanted to be able to drive. Working with red and green glasses made it possible for me to have partial three-dimensional vision and to eventually see well enough to start learning to drive and to know where I was on the road.

You may not have such a dramatic change, but having better three-dimensional vision and having a distinction between the two eyes is a great way to reduce your cross-sightedness.

Object and Line

The first step is to make a division between the two eyes completely and to unite them in the brain. Wearing the red and green glasses, you may see light with one eye and an object with the other. Some people will not see light or an object. The aim of this exercise is to get both eyes working together.

For this exercise you will need a red pen or pencil, a piece of white paper, and a small flashlight with a red bulb. If you don't have a red bulb, put some red masking tape over the flashlight lens to simulate a red filter.

Draw a red circle on the white sheet of paper. Hold the paper out in front of you with one hand so that the paper is parallel to the ground, about a foot in front of your eyes. Turn the flashlight on and put it underneath the paper, shining the light up through it. Look down at the circle while shining the light up through the page. You should see the circle and also the light.

Now close your red-filtered eye. The eye that looks through the green filter should see the circle but not the light, because the red light cannot penetrate through the green lens. On the other hand, the green filter does not stop you from seeing the red circle.

Conversely, if you close the eye that looks through the green, and only look through the red lens, you will see the light, but you will not see the red circle. The eye with the green filter will only see the object, and the eye with the red filter will only see the light. This kind of division is very important because you see a separate image from the eye with the red filter and the eye with the green filter simultaneously.

Now move the light, which is underneath the page, around the perimeter of the circle, like you are tracing around its edge. If your eyes can track together, you will be able to keep the light on the edge of the circle. If your eyes cannot track together, though you may think that the light is on the edge of the circle, it will actually be elsewhere. In my case, when I thought that the light was on the circle, the light was actually outside or inside the circle. So, a way for you to know what's happening with your light is to suddenly close the eye with the green filter; when you do this, you will see exactly where the light is. When you open the eye with the green filter, you will see if the light remains exactly where it was when that eye was closed, or if it moved. Even if it moved, don't correct it. Close your eye with the green lens and open it ten to twenty times or until the

light remains in the same place as it does when you look at the light through the red lens alone. Once it stays in the same place, it means that your eyes are tracking. For it doesn't matter if it's in the circle or out; what matters is that the two eyes are looking together at the same spot.

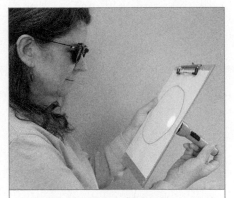

You may find yourself needing to palm in the middle of this exercise. Palm for as long as necessary to help you relax enough to return to the exercise.

Figure 5.6. Turn the flashlight on and put it underneath the paper, shining the light up through it.

Now change the glasses. That is, if you first put the red lens on the left eye and the green on the right eye, now put the green on the left eye and the red on the right eye; then repeat the exercise.

Another exercise you can do with the red and green glasses is to have someone draw a line with the red pencil, and you try to trace the line with a red pencil while wearing the red filter over your strong eye. The reason for this is that through the red lens you will not be able to see red lines or red writing (unless you are in the 2 percent of the population who can see a red line or red writing through a red lens, in which case the other exercises are more appropriate for you).

You will want to put the red lens in front of the strong eye so the weaker eye will read the red print, but the stronger eye will not read the red line or print. The two eyes will see most other colors together, but the eye with the red filter won't be able to see whatever is red, and that changes domination for a moment, which could be five to eight minutes. The weaker eye will take a front seat, and, as a result, the brain will learn to use it more in your day-to-day activity.

A variation of this exercise is to take some white paper, wear the red lens in front of the strong eye, and write in big letters anything you like, for example, your name and four other names of people familiar to you on one page and a few words of a poem that you like on another. Then trace what you wrote and see if you can match the original writing.

Card Game

This is a fun and effective way to help balance the two eyes because you don't even realize that you're doing an exercise, and you create body/eye coordination as well. Let's say the left eye is weaker; it will now have to work no less than the right eye, which has no control over it in this situation.

You start off with a special deck of cards (two decks, if you have a few people playing) specifically designed to work with the red and green glasses. The deck is made up of two different colored cards: half the deck is red with black letters, and the other half is white with red letters. You

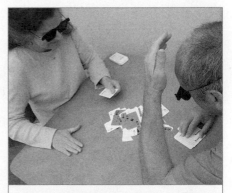

Figure 5.7. Playing a variation of the card game War.

can only see the white cards with the green lens and the red cards with the red lens. As this game proceeds, you and others wear the glasses while you each simultaneously throw down a card from your own portion of the deck. When you identify certain numbers, you will react with a corresponding physical response. For instance, when you see a card with a nine on it, you clap your hands; when you see a seven, you tap your forehead; when you see an ace, you stamp on the floor and bang on the table, etc. The responses could match whatever four cards you would like them to match, and could be anything you are able to dream up. The point is to do something with your body in response to the numbers you have designated in the cards. The person who reacts the quickest when one of these cards is thrown is the one who gets to keep the pile. When it appears that about half of the cards have been thrown, reverse your glasses so that each eye has a chance to see through both the red filter and the green filter.

It's better, and more fun, to have two or three people playing this game along with you. Extra pairs of glasses are inexpensive and can be purchased at the School for Self-Healing, as can the cards themselves. As enjoyable as it is, this game has had significant results: there has been a temporary improvement in the vision of 50 percent of the people who have played it.

Chapter 6

Pathology Conditions

Correcting Cataracts

A cataract, put simply, is a cloudy spot on the lens of the eye. One theory is that cataracts are the result of a crowding of proteins within the lens, which prevents light from passing through. This in turn causes an obstruction that eventually makes vision blur or can make a person completely blind.

Since the purpose of the lens is to transfer light to the retina, you can see why a cloudy spot on the lens would make seeing difficult. Most people experience fuzziness of vision when they reach their mid-sixties to midseventies. Upon visits to their eye doctors, they discover that they have cataracts.

There are quite a few reasons for cataracts, including poor nutrition and poor metabolism in the body. It is important, therefore, to eat a balanced, healthy diet and to devote time to regular exercise, especially as we get older.

Many other reasons for cataracts are unknown, and in fact most people don't really care what the cause of their cataract is because the medical solution seems to work fine for most people, which is simply to remove the lens. Cataracts occur so regularly that we think it is natural, and there is no way to stop it or to save the lens. If the lens is removed surgically and an intraocular lens is inserted artificially, most people regain the vast majority of their vision. After all, you do not see with your lens—you see with your retina and your brain.

In fact, that tends to be the treatment we like these days. We like to remove parts that are not essential to our daily functions and either replace them or live without them; then we hail conventional medicine for being able to do it. While I'm happy that cataract surgeries exist (especially because some people cannot manage their cataracts, and the lens needs to be removed anyway), I would like to propose that in 80 percent of the cases when cataracts begin, they can be stalled and even stopped for dozens of years, if not eliminated altogether. Moreover, cataracts can be prevented. The lens of modern life does not have the chance for full functioning. It becomes thick and opaque because it doesn't move the way it was designed by nature to move.

With the exception a child whose lens is opaque in infancy, in which case medicine has proven to be a great relief to many children, we need to fight for every lens when cataracts begin. My feeling is that if we did this, most of the people destined for cataract surgery these days would never actually have it. Often, surgery makes the eyes even worse because it causes scar tissue to build up on the lens. Other times, we have glaucoma attacks that could blind the eye, or there is bleeding in the retina as a result of cataract surgery.

One of my patients, Brett, had diabetes. His left eye was operated on successfully and was at 20/20 vision. When his right eye was operated on, he became blind. I had partial success with Brett's right eye using light therapy, but his doctor negated the results, and Brett lost the small progress he had made with me. Doctors' suggestions can be very powerful. For that reason, I failed in my therapy with Brett, and it was heartbreaking because I liked this wonderful person, and I wanted very much to succeed with him.

On the other hand, one of my best friends and clients, Hannan, had one eye that was sighted and the other nearly blind. We worked for ten years and were able to get the blind eye to see somewhat and the sighted eye to see better than he had seen since childhood.

Then Hannan went to Bascom Palmer, one of the best hospitals in the United States, and had cataract surgery. There were complications in the surgery itself. But after the four-hour surgery that should have lasted for only forty minutes, his vision became 20/25, 95 percent of 20/20, to the amazement of all attending physicians.

We never know what's going to be the result of a medical procedure. Sometimes it's worse than we imagine it would be, as with Brett, who had expected to see 20/20 in his right eye. Brett's doctors didn't take into consideration that his calf had to be amputated from the knee down due to diabetes-related gangrene and that his circulation couldn't possibly be the same when they operated on his right eye. Therefore, the result of the surgery in his right eye was not nearly as positive as it was in the previous surgery in his left eye. But in Hannan's case, where the physicians were sure there would not be any good results from the surgery, it was Hannan's insistence that caused them to do the surgery after the cataract was in place for a great many years. He ended up seeing 20/25.

What an amazing dichotomy: when they expect to succeed, they fail; when they expect to fail, they succeed.

When one eye overworks and the other eye underworks because of a cataract, the brain works very hard to suppress the information that the underworking eye brings to it. The strain is immeasurable. The eye that overworks becomes fatigued; the eye that underworks becomes weak.

If you experience a cataract, my advice is simply to work on yourself, first with the exercises recommended in this chapter. Remember to refer back to Chapter 4 for specific instructions for each exercise. The goal is to get both eyes to work together and to get the weaker eye to pull its fair share and not get dominated by the stronger eye. Only if your self-care fails to achieve the desired results should you seek help from surgeons.

Exercise Program for Cataracts

- Look into the Distance: 30 minutes daily, three intervals of 10 minutes, or 20 minutes once and 10 minutes once.
- Look at Details: 10 minutes daily.
- Palming: 60 minutes daily.
- Bounce and Catch: 10 minutes daily.

A Note about Cataract Surgery

If you are considering cataract surgery, the purpose of doing these exercises is to see whether you can postpone or even cancel the surgery. When you do this program, you should ask yourself if you are improving. If you are, postpone the surgery.

Many people have improved or have halted the onset of cataracts, so they didn't need the surgery. Some, however, have not improved. But even for those who did not improve, the fact that they did the exercises was good anyway. So don't stop the exercises even if you did not succeed in stopping the cataract.

These exercises are good for the overall health of the eye. That is your goal. The goal isn't to avoid surgery; it is the health of the eye. If you can prevent the surgery, that's great, and that happens to more than half of the people who follow this program.

We work very hard from infancy to early childhood to create balanced use of the two eyes. Pediatric ophthalmologists understand how important it is to create bilateral vision. What puzzles me, however, is that most ophthalmologists will correct one eye to see near with cataract surgery and one eye to see far. This correction is an error, and it goes completely against nature's will for the eyes to work together. It strains the eye and creates tension all over the body.

The best solution is to request that your surgeon correct both eyes to see well from far away, and with glasses to see well from close up. With time and exercise, maybe you won't need the glasses.

Note: Remember to work these exercises into the entirety of your day. Don't do an hour and a half all at once. Pace out the exercises so that you are working on your vision all the time, as a matter of habit. Habits determine your destiny.

Extra Exercise for Cataracts: Bounce and Catch

For this exercise you will need the opaque piece of paper to tape to the bridge of your nose, a ball, and, if possible, a trampoline. If you are not able to find a trampoline, or if your physical condition prevents you from using one, you can simply try running in place instead of bouncing. The point of bouncing is to distract your mind and body while you practice the exercise, as well as to engage your peripheral and central vision in a dynamic and different way.

Simply put the paper on the bridge of your nose so it blocks the central vision of the strong eye, and play catch with someone while you bounce. Wave one hand to the side, above, and also below the eye that is obstructed. Make sure that you can see your hand only peripherally. Bounce and catch for five minutes; then take a break and sun for a minute. Then bounce and catch for another five minutes. Now take the piece of paper off and see how different the world looks. Notice a bigger periphery expanding around you. Notice the intensity of color and shape. It is also helpful to try this exercise with the paper taped to the bridge of your nose from your forehead down to your chin, as in the Melissa exercise.

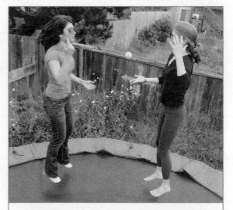

Figure 6.1. The point of bouncing is to distract your mind and body while you practice the exercise.

Correcting Diabetes

Diabetes is a condition caused when the body cannot produce insulin or does not utilize insulin in the right way. Insulin is actually a hormone. Insulin's basic function is to transfer sugar (glucose) into the body's cells. There is also a tendency for patients with diabetes to experience poor blood flow.

Poor blood flow can lead to major difficulties in the body, from heart problems to a loss of limbs. And today, we are very aware of how important proper blood flow is to the visual system. Because of poor blood flow to the eyes, some diabetic patients get cataracts, retinopathy, and neovascularization, which are very similar to conditions related to high blood pressure. They lead to continuous bleeding in the retina, which could lead to blindness.

Poor blood flow leads to a response in the retina in which new vesicles are formed. This response is very useful in every other part of the body. For example, if you are bedridden for a month because of a serious illness, you'll have pain when you first stand up, partly because you don't have enough blood flow to your legs. Very quickly, though, the body will form capillaries to bring you circulation, sometimes called *collateral circulation.* If your main arteries are clogged or not functional in any way, when the main arteries open up, those vesicles (the capillaries) will degenerate, and the main blood vessels will take over. So, the second or third time that you stand, your legs won't hurt.

Because of diabetes, high blood pressure, or other systemic problems, you do not get enough blood flow to the retina, and the body will form capillaries to nourish the retina. Many times those capillaries are defective; they leak and destroy the sensitive and small photoreceptive cells.

To prevent diabetic attacks, always carry fruits or seeds wherever you go so you can have healthy snacks if there is a rise in your sugar level. More important, learn to exercise in a way that loosens the neck and brings more blood flow to your whole body and prevents lack of blood flow to your head and retinas.

Exercise Program for Diabetes: 40 Minutes Daily

- Massage: 20 minutes daily.
- Shifting/Looking at Details: 10 minutes daily.
- Extra Exercise for Diabetes: 10 minutes daily.

Many people with diabetes do not develop eye problems. Doing these specific exercises may help the health of the eye. Concentrating on neck and shoulder exercises may prevent eye problems from occurring because what we need is more blood flow.

Incorporate these exercises into every part of your day. Don't just practice for one hour in the morning or one hour at night.

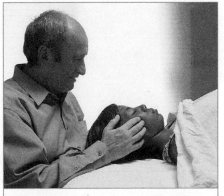

Figure 6.2. Bringing more blood flow to the head and retinas.

Find five minutes here and five minutes there, all day, every day. Your diabetes is with you every minute of the day. So you must work to overcome the disadvantages of your diabetes constantly.

For your extra daily exercise, you may choose from any of the following. On some days you might want to practice them all!

Extra Exercises for Diabetes

Tapping

I have found throughout the years that tapping on all the bones of the body makes a difference with diabetes. After massaging your face, head, eyes, neck, and shoulders, tap rapidly with your fingertips on every bone of your body. You can also stand under the shower and have the shower massager tap on every single bone of your body.

Tapping helps to stimulate blood production.

It's also good for you to sit down, hold your legs, and rub your feet one against the other. That can help you to create more circulation. The extremities, such as the feet and hands, are far from the heart. So are the face and, of course, the eyes, and they have a complex vascular system as well. What we want is to bring better blood flow to every part of the body. Blood flow is what nurtures the body. The better the blood flow, the more vital, vibrant, and happy we become.

Whenever you massage your body, you have to massage toward the heart. Start by massaging your feet, then your calves, and then your thighs in a rotating motion. Then massage your buttocks with your palms; use your fingertips to massage your inguinal area to loosen up the tension in the hips. Then massage your abdominal area firmly, but with some gentleness, and in a rotating motion toward the heart. Massage your chest and tap on the bones in your chest. Next, massage your forehead and then your entire head. This massage therapy can make a very big difference in terms of the blood flow in your body.

Waving

Many people with diabetes develop a major blind spot in their retina. If this is happening to you, hang an eye chart on the wall at eye level and wave your hand in the area of the blind spot while looking with the healthy areas at the eye chart.

For this exercise, the point is to go back and do all the other eye chart exercises while waving your hand in the area of the blind spot you are experiencing. Review all the exercises in the rest of the book and do them with the stronger eye while you wave your hand in the blind spot.

Patch the Strong Eye

If you have a small damaged portion in one of your retinas, wear a patch on your strong eye and place a piece of paper with a small opening in the area of blindness in front of your weaker eye. Then go for a walk around your yard or somewhere else safe. This will force the weakest part of your eye to do all the work.

If you cannot see anything this way, go into a dark room with your strong eye patched and put blinking lights in front of the weak eye until you begin to experience some sensation of light in the blind spot. Refer to the chapter on glaucoma for suggestions on using blinking lights.

A Note about Laser Treatments

I would like to discourage you from having too many laser treatments. Many concerned physicians do preventive laser treatments in which they basically scar a big portion of the retina to prevent rubeosis, or bleeding in the retina. But if you improve your blood flow, there will be no rubeosis.

Too many laser treatments can weaken the retina and blind too many parts of it. So while I respect and accept the use of laser treatments to stop continuous bleeding once it occurs, I would like you to aggressively embrace exercises, movement, and dietary change and to work on damaged areas in order to help the parts that are not damaged.

These days, doctors use injections to stop bleeding. While injections of Lucentis and other future medications may be effective and less damaging than laser treatments, they still have some damaging effects. My recommendation is to do the injections only when there is bleeding, and not otherwise. Exercise to increase the blood flow, and you will decrease the bleeding.

Cataracts and Diabetes

If you do have cataract surgery, pay attention to your general blood flow and demand to be checked by the doctor every two hours after the surgery. Doctors hate to be patronized by patients, but don't worry about it. Your health comes first. Make sure that you are being tested every two hours, and have them test you for bleeding and for any compromise of your retina or optic nerve.

Correcting Glaucoma

Glaucoma is a disease of the optic nerve, often caused by irregular pressure in the eyes, that results in loss of the visual field and, eventually, blindness. Glaucoma can be a scary disease for many people because of this, and also since its symptoms may not be obvious until the disease is quite advanced.

The loss of vision that occurs with glaucoma has a few factors. One is pressure, and another is weakness of the optic nerve and disk (the area where the nerve connects to the retina). So if you have a very strong optic nerve and disk, even high pressure will not necessarily lead to a loss of vision. But if you have a weak optic nerve and disk, even low pressure could lead to a loss of vision. For this reason, everyone must be evaluated to determine whether they have a weak or a strong optic nerve and disk before the effects of pressure can be understood and predicted accurately.

The complication here comes from Lasik surgery because it alters the thickness of the cornea, which will alter the perception of pressure, thus making it harder to measure. To date, it has been difficult to determine what the pressure truly is after Lasik surgery.

We would like to assume that normal pressure in the eye is between 10 and 20 mercury points. Anything less than 10 could be insufficient pressure on the eye. We need pressure in the eye just like a tire needs pressure to maintain its integrity. But when the pressure mounts, it can destroy weak areas in our eyes. The main area that it destroys is the optic disk, which is rather weak in all of us but is even weaker in people who have glaucoma. Reducing pressure would take away the risk of blindness or, at least, of partial blindness.

Statistically, it is true to say that those who have pressure above 30 will most likely lose more vision, but only statistically. In any particular case, it could be that even a pressure higher than 30 does not lead to vision loss. You could also say that some people at a pressure of only 24 or 25 may lose a lot of vision.

The other problem that could easily occur is low-tension glaucoma. With low-tension glaucoma, the optic disk degenerates and is destroyed even at a pressure under that which is considered to be desirable for most of us. The optic disk is a weak and vulnerable area. When that area has pressure it cannot withstand, the optic disk can be compromised. In some people with completely normal pressure (the 16 mercury points that most of us would desire to have), the optic disk can still be destroyed. Still, the prevailing viewpoint is that the problem is the high pressure in high-tension glaucoma patients, and if they have surgery to reduce the pressure, the problems will go away. While I agree with it to a point, I believe that it is only a part of what happens. Therefore, the treatment is sometimes ineffective, and can even be dangerous because it works only on the eye pressure without considering other factors.

Recently I had the pleasure of working with a bright woman named Lucia, who came all the way from Brazil to San Francisco for two weeks of intensive sessions with me. She came to me with much fear because she had lost 95 percent of her nerve functionality due to glaucoma. The surprising thing about her case was that, after doing the eye exercises and before she even met with me, she gained back the peripheral vision she had lost; her field of vision was almost completely normal—there was only one small spot of vision loss—and her acuity was 20/20. I am not the only one who is surprised with such magnificent vision after such significant loss of nerve tissue.

Lucia also told me that several of her family members were afflicted with cardiovascular disease. Knowing that she had this family history, my conclusion from her case was that doing the exercises had increased her blood flow to the remaining nerve tissue and had improved the situation tremendously. Doctors had offered her a very risky surgery to reduce the pressure, but it would have also posed a big risk to her vision, and she could have lost it completely. I am happy she refused.

I believe that the following can help people with glaucoma:

- Reduction of pressure (in this I agree with doctors)
- Balanced use of the two eyes and within each eye
- Sufficient circulation to nourish the optic nerve

In Lucia's case, the bodywork we did was just as important as the vision work, and the part of the nerve that was working assumed the work of the nerves that had been destroyed.

The frustrating part of it all is that even when you reduce the pressure to 10 or 11, as many doctors want you to do, the optic disk may be fine but could also continue to erode to the point of destruction, causing damage to the optic nerve. And the feeling shared by medical doctors is that the optic nerve can never regenerate.

Unlike cataract surgery, about which physicians are very optimistic, physicians continuously see that they cannot fully control glaucoma: not with drops, not with surgery. There is no way to clarify to anyone that reduction of pressure equals reduction of destruction of the optic nerve. And it is clear that most people like to have a simple technical solution to complex problems. Since there seems to be no magic bullet for glaucoma, people live in fear. And that fear is one of the main destructive dangers to our eyes.

The eyes feel this fear. The tissues feel the fear as well, and then become much worse. With some of my patients who had temporary improvement in therapy, I sometimes felt that this cloud of fear caused them to deteriorate anyway. With other patients, where the situation seemed to be grave to everyone else, their trust in the therapy dramatically improved their vision through the correct exercises and the right knowledge. Positive affirmation can be very useful. You can close your eyes and visualize that the strength of your eyes outpowers any phenomenon that can destroy them. Positive affirmation is 50 percent of your healing process.

When it comes to high pressure in the eyes, all factors must be considered: lack of balanced use of the eyes, stiffness of the neck (which is a result of stiffness of the body), or even a sense of emotional loss—not just stress, but loss.

A good example is the desire for peace and harmony in a relationship, but never finding it because of resolutions that never come. Similarly, kids of divorced parents feel this when they want to see their parents getting along but never do. There are many different situations that can cause glaucoma, so apply this book in a way that works for your specific situation.

Some people may have lost a lot of vision before the practice of these exercises and will do anything they can to keep the vision they already have and to sharpen it to a great extent. Other people may have lost hardly any vision and, therefore, do the eye exercises to prevent any potential vision loss and to sharpen their vision. Some people may have only a mild vision loss. Pay attention to the area where your vision is mildly lost, and use the area that is fuzzy or almost blind; this will help you to defend the rest of your visual system. So, apply the book individually to your needs. Take time and pay attention to yourself in a way that works for you.

I will never forget one of my dearest patients, Murray, who had glaucoma. He did well in his therapy with me for a period of seven years. But he took a turn for the worse when his wife died. Issues between him and his wife were never resolved, and that's one of the worst situations when a person you love perishes. If a person who was very dear to you did not get along with you, and the problem you had with that person was never resolved, with their death comes a sense of loss without closure. Part of this loss is not processing your inner feelings around the unresolved issues you had with the deceased. Murray had a problem with his wife's senility and the Alzheimer's she had developed toward the end of her life. He discovered much anger that she had against some people which she had never brought out during their marital life. It revealed much of her anguish that he had never noticed during her youth. He was struck by the amount of anger and frustration that came out of her when she forgot the present and only remembered the past. And here was a woman who was a world educator and a writer.

When she died, his glaucoma became much worse because his emotional state lacked the stability that he had during most of the marriage. He was also exhausted from trying to keep his wife in as good a shape as he could during the last years of her life. Often, when there is a sense of loss and death, it can lead to a loss of vision. A sense of loss or death could result from the absence of anything that you really loved and adored, like relationships, stability, or a home you had liked but from which you had to move. Anything that deep inside leads to an emotional connection, and when it leaves your life without a positive resolution, it could lead to tremendous subconscious tension. That tension reveals itself as a great muscular contraction in your neck. And that neck contraction hampers and disturbs the blood flow to your brain and to your eyes. When it disturbs the blood flow to your brain, you run a risk of strokes and hemorrhages of the brain cells. When it disturbs the blood flow to your eyes, you run the risk of losing retinal areas and vision, and you run a greater risk of having high pressure in your eyes.

Exercise Program for Glaucoma

- Peripheral Exercise: 20 minutes daily.
- Palming: 6 minutes at a time, three times daily, with at least 5 minutes between sessions for 30 minutes a day.
- Sunning: 20 minutes daily.
- Headlines (from the section on astigmatism): 10 minutes.
- Block the Strong Eye (tape the medium-sized piece of paper onto the bridge of your nose so that it blocks the central vision of your strong eye; now read with your weaker eye while waving your hand in the periphery of your stronger eye): 10 minutes.
- Physical Exercises for Glaucoma: 20 minutes daily.

Note: While working on your eyes, also address your emotional state and create a good emotional environment for yourself. And remember to work on your eyes throughout the day. Find time here and there to always work on healing your vision.

Physical Exercises for Glaucoma

Good thoughts and good prayer can be healing. Visualize that blood is circulating to your retina, making it soft and nurturing your optic disk. Also visualize that the fluid in its clear form is flowing in the area between the cornea and the macula. Visualize that good blood circulation is nourishing your optic disk and retina. Visualize the blood coming from the back, and from your neck to the back of the head, and nourishing your optic disk. Visualize that blood is flowing into your eye and draining from it. Then visualize that the aqueous humor is flowing into the front area of your eye from the lens to the cornea, nourishing both, and draining into the area of your nose. It's amazing how powerful the body is and how much it does all at once. It's not power that belongs to you but to nature, and you are a wonderful guest of nature's within your own body. There is a connection between that power and of all universal powers around you; this connection gives that power a tremendous amount of strength.

The power that brings rain from the sky and wind to the earth, the power that is mysterious to all of us and runs the whole universe, is the same power that moves your blood and your fluids. It does so constantly. The more you acknowledge its power and its strength, the better it will work for you. There is a connection between your mind and soul and the natural functions of your body. When you have glaucoma, physical exercises are important to prevent the pressure from mounting and growing in your eyes and, in fact, will reduce it. Other exercises will be important to preserve your vision. All of them will be a pleasure to do. When you work on your body, you work for the purpose of having fun with it, and it is a pleasure to do the work. When you have that feeling, it's going to be wonderful to heal your glaucoma and to overcome it. It will create a better connection between you and your internal forces, and it will help you to tune in to the forces of the universe. It's probably the best antidepressant you can ever have.

Special Instructions for Palming with Glaucoma

You should only palm for up to ten minutes at a time. Then wait at least five minutes before palming again. You can do this many times a day. But if you palm too long all in one session, you can experience an increase in pressure. If, for example, you have closed-angle glaucoma and you palm for a half an hour all at once, you can have an increase in pressure of 4 mercury points.

Exercises for Glaucoma

Sunning is one of the best eye exercises you can do for glaucoma because it temporarily reduces your pressure. It also contracts the pupils and creates better fluid flow within your eyes. So, for the time that you do it, your pressure is being reduced. And the reduction of pressure will last if you could also release the tension in your neck. This exercise will help you do that.

If you are a typical glaucoma patient, if such a thing exists, most likely you have a very tight neck. Tension of the neck, to a great extent, is a result of mental stress as well as physical stress, but not in all cases. Nevertheless, I have found that many people who have a tendency for glaucoma exacerbate that tendency with either injury or tension in the neck.

It's important for you to know that you need to work on your neck, first spiritually, then mentally. It's good to write about your thoughts and feelings in a journal. Then meet with a good friend or maybe with a psychotherapist who can help you. Hopefully, with holistic inclinations, you will see your whole life and all phenomena as one unified experience.

Sometimes, it's important for you to take a good vacation or to do things that can improve your life. For example, let yourself be drawn into having a relationship if you don't have one, or into finding a way to get out of your shell of loneliness if you are lonely. And, if you have a relationship, allow yourself to examine it and to find out if you really spend enough time with your partner; allow yourself to develop good communication skills with your partner in order to bring smoothness into your life. It's important to do the work that will help you to feel that you are doing well emotionally and that you're advancing yourself spiritually. Then, you just may find yourself in a whole new place of physical self-improvement with these exercises. Often, the exercises will bring back emotional phenomena, which you'll want to deal with whenever they come, in order to reach a place of neutrality and tranquility.

These days, many people do not understand the value of neutrality. Somebody wrote me a postcard that said, "Meir, never tell me to relax. My tension is the only thing that holds me together." That's why many people function with tremendous amounts of tension and think it's good: because they always have it. Life is much happier with less tension. In a place of relaxation, you feel security and love in the universe.

Now, while facing the sun with your eyes closed, hold your head steady and stroke your cheekbones, massaging around your eyes and nose. Massaging the areas around your eyes is very helpful for relaxation. Quite often, the tension of the eyes leads to squinting, as I've mentioned throughout this book. That is a tension that you want to undo. When you take away squinting, you take away pressure, and when you take away pressure, the eye becomes healthy.

Move your head from side to side. Then move your head up and down while moving from side to side. Your chin points up toward the sky and down toward your chest. You should move your head up and down four times, from the edge of your shoulder to the middle, and four times from the middle of your shoulder to the edge. This really helps to loosen up your neck and to create more space between the first vertebrae and the crown. After doing this forty times, palm for thirty seconds. Then you should do it another forty times, if you can relax while performing the exercise. Do not massage around the eyes here, because it's not safe to do this when you move the head up and down. Just move your head up and down as you're facing the sun with your eyes closed. Then palm again. Do this exercise a third time and then palm yet again for thirty seconds to a minute. Next, move your head from side to side and massage your eyebrows and cheekbones.

Now bend your knees and straighten them again. Try to bring your knees to the level of your abdomen or chest (this depends on how flexible your hips are) while moving the head from side to side. If balance is an issue, hold onto a wall or a chair as you do this exercise. Make sure that you don't fall while doing it.

Now march in place and move your head from side to side while moving your legs from side to side in order to pump more blood into the head and loosen the neck. If you have good balance, then as you move your legs up and down and move your head from side to side, massage your hands. Especially massage the place in the palm that is between the thumb and the second finger. If it's hard for you to do three things at once (moving your head from side to side all the way gently and steadily, moving your legs up and down, and massaging your palm, all at the same time), then you can do two things. Massage your hand and move your head from side to side, or move your head from side to side and just move your legs up and down. Those are things that can help you to bring more blood flow and to calm your nervous system; don't strain to do them.

After massaging your palm, and while moving your legs up and down, just simply move your head from side to side twenty or thirty times; then go indoors and palm for eight minutes. When you relax from the palming, you will have time to loosen up your neck.

Before doing neck exercises, determine how well your neck moves from side to side. Once you have an idea of the range of motion available to you, begin these exercises so that, at first, you stay within your comfortable range of motion. Gradually, this range of motion should increase over time. Also, with all these neck exercises, you should strive for fifteen to twenty repetitions on each side for each exercise.

Now lie on your back, bend your knees, stretch your arms, and look at one hand; let's say the right hand. Take the left hand and bring it all the way to the right and, in fact, surpass it. Stay there for one deep breath. Keep your head looking at the right while bringing the left hand all the way to the left. The shoulder will then stretch in two ways. For one, it will stretch in the back muscles, the trapezius and the rhomboids, in order to bring the arm forward. The second time, when you bring your arm back to where it was, the pectoral muscles of the chest will stretch, and the chest muscles as well as the back muscles are directly connected to neck muscles.

Then move your head to the opposite side and do exactly the same exercise with your right hand reaching to the left. You can let your legs move after your arm if that's what your body needs to do to complete

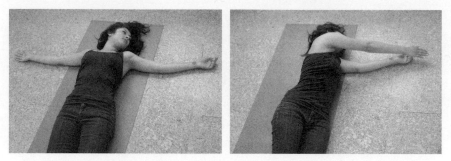

Figure 6.3. (a) Bend your knees, stretch out your arms, and turn to face your left hand. (b) Reach your right arm across to and past the left hand.

the stretch. Repeat the exercise thirty-five times. Then move your head from side to side; 90 percent of people feel that the neck is looser when they do this exercise. Then put your hands behind your head and lift up your head without the neck helping you. Do this six or seven times. See if you can let go of your neck and just let your hands do the work. Then put one hand on your forehead and move your head from side to side, with your hand on your forehead and your neck loosening.

Another great exercise for the neck is to walk backward. Do that for 400 or 500 yards a day, every day. Look over your shoulder from time to time, which is also a great exercise to stretch your neck. At the same time, it's good for you to work with a friend, at least once a week, although a few times a week is even better. While you lie on the floor, your friend will put his or her legs on your shoulders to hold you in place, put one hand cupped under your chin and the other cupped at the occipital bone, and gently pull, stretching and elongating your neck.

Another wonderful exercise for the neck is to sit on a chair, put your chin on your chest, and then slowly bend down until you touch the floor. Then straighten up with your legs first, and then with your whole back. Now do the same thing from a standing position. Bend over, putting your chin on your chest, and slowly bend down, vertebra by vertebra. Put your hand on the floor and, only after you do, sit on the chair while still bending. Then, keeping your chin on your chest and your hands on the floor, you straighten.

Next, if you do not have a tendency for retinal detachment, which many people with glaucoma do not, you can also sit cross-legged and move your whole body in a rotating motion. Sit on the floor with your legs crossed. Put your hands on your knees. Now bend forward and rotate your whole body in a broad circular motion, bending at the waist, rotating all the way around one way and then the other, feeling your spine elongate and your neck stretch. Go both directions: left, then right. Now put both hands on the right leg and lean forward so that your forehead touches your right knee. Lean forward, then straighten back up. Do this five times. Then put both hands on your left knee. Bend forward so your forehead touches your left knee, then straighten back up. Do this five times. Now bend at the waist and rotate your whole body again.

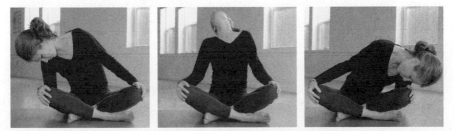

Figure 6.4. (a) Also sit cross-legged and move your whole body in a rotating motion. (b) Let the head roll loosely as your body rotates. (c) Make big, full circles with your body.

Next (as long as you don't have retinal detachment), get down on all fours and put the crown of your head on the floor. Rotate your head to the left and to the right, keeping your forehead in contact with the floor. Go right and left slowly, gently breathing in and out. Now, keeping the crown of your head in contact with the floor, rotate your head in a circular motion on the floor. You might just feel your scalp coming to life! Move the crown of your head on the floor, in a rotating motion, breathing deeply and slowly. If this hurts, simply modify the pressure on your head by using your hands to support your weight. Go back to sitting cross-legged again and move your body once more in a rotating motion, bending at the waist. Take your time and breathe. Really feel how relaxed your neck is becoming.

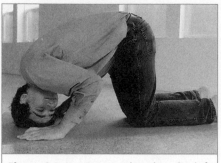

Figure 6.5. Rotate your head to the left and to the right several times and then in a circular motion on the floor.

Next you will want to sit down on the floor with your back against a wall and your knees bent in front of you. If for any reason (i.e., a very large belly) you have a hard time bending your knees, sit cross-legged instead. Otherwise, bend your knees. If you want, you can put a small pillow behind the middle of your back, underneath the shoulders, to make it more comfortable.

First move your head all the way to the left so that you are stretching your neck muscles as you breathe deeply. Tap your fingers on the stretched muscles on the opposite side of your neck. Massage the neck muscles with your thumb and fingers. Now turn your head in the other direction, stretching the other side of your neck, and do the same thing on the opposite side, tapping the stretched muscles with your fingers and then massaging that side of the neck with your thumb and fingers.

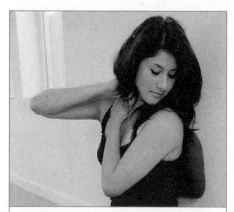

Figure 6.6. Tap your fingers on the stretched muscles on the opposite side of your neck.

After several repetitions on both sides, interlace your fingers underneath your knees and bend forward so your forehead touches your knees about twenty times, which loosens up the middle of your back.

Put your hands on your knees and push your legs to one side and then the other, using only the strength of your hands, not your legs. Push your knees to the left and then to the right. You will feel yourself starting to scoot forward and to slip down on the wall; that's okay. Just pause and scoot yourself back up into the seated position with which you had started. Start over again from the beginning, turning your head from side to side. You may find that your neck is much looser now.

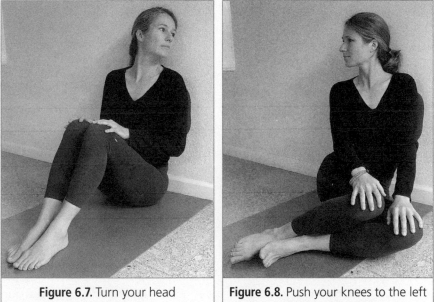

Figure 6.7. Turn your head from side to side. **Figure 6.8.** Push your knees to the left and then to the right.

It's also a very good idea to close your eyes and to put a warm towel over them. Moisten the towel with warm water or with herbal tea; Eye Bright tea, in particular, has been very effective for me.

Another thing that my clients like very much is the steam machine that my sister, who owns health spas, has donated to our school. Steam in a dark room can be very relaxing when you have your eyes closed.

These exercises are essential for reduction of tension. After doing these exercises every day for a period of time of around three months, measure your pressure and see if it has gone down. If so, you may be able to prevent the need to use eye drops, as long as your ophthalmologist does not oppose the idea; at the very least you may be able to reduce them gradually with supervision. Find a friendly ophthalmologist or optometrist who is willing to measure your pressure frequently, ideally twice a week, so you will know that you are on the right path.

Correcting Optic Neuritis

Optic neuritis is a condition caused by a temporary swelling from inflammation of the optic nerve. The worst-case scenario with optic neuritis is that less blood will flow to the optic nerve; because of poor blood flow, there will be ischemia of the nerve, a part of which could degenerate and wither.

In most cases optic neuritis comes and goes. Physicians believe they can help this condition with steroid treatments. Sometimes, the steroid treatments work, and the optic neuritis does not return frequently. At other times, however, the treatments create dependency.

When you suffer from optic neuritis, a very good thing is to spend a lot of time in a completely dark room. This gives your whole body, as well as your eyes, a great chance to relax. By far the best solution for optic neuritis is a long session of palming. This is true whether the cause is the optic nerve itself or a systemic illness like multiple sclerosis that impacts many other nerves besides the optic nerve.

Imagine that you walk a lot and step on your legs in an imbalanced way. Consequently, you would develop swelling in your legs. Physicians would correctly tell you to rest your leg, maybe to put a brace or a bandage on your ankle or, perhaps, to use crutches. Any of the those would be intended to give your leg the rest it needs to heal so that it can return to its proper functioning. In many ways, the same approach is good for the optic nerve. You must rest your optic nerve for the inflammation of the nerve to disappear.

Staying in a dark room and covering your eyes with a light cloth for a day, or perhaps two days, and not walking much in daylight could be the best solution for optic neuritis. It's also good to massage your neck and your back.

This is a very important piece of information for millions of people. No one gives you the suggestion to lie and rest in the dark. Hospital rooms are fully lit all the time for the purpose of security and control. Lack of darkness in hospital rooms can exacerbate a problem like this. Being at home in the most familiar surroundings can make a difference, especially with fresh air and loving palms over your closed eyes to give you a sense of nurturing. When you lie in the dark with your eyes closed, or when you sit in the dark and palm, you allow for complete replenishment of the optic nerve, which is more important than any medication you can possibly get.

Medication can help in extreme cases, but sometimes it produces terrible side effects. Sitting in the dark has helped the majority of my clients who have had different attacks of optic neuritis. I advise the clients with whom I work in person that only if this doesn't work should medication become an option. Since you, the reader, are not working with me in person, I advise you to work with a physician who is not opposed to your self-healing practices. Be sure, as you follow my recommendations, to consult with a trusted physician, one who knows your condition well and to whom you have easy access during this process. This would determine the urgency, or not, for you to be put on medication.

When the optic neuritis passes, diligently practice the ten steps in Chapter 2.

Correcting Detached Retinas and Retinal Tears

A detached retina is a very serious problem that almost always causes partial or full blindness unless it is treated.

The retina performs a function similar to the film in a camera. Located in the back of the eye, it receives optical images, converts them to chemical reactions, and transmits them through the optic nerve to the brain for interpretation.

The retina is considered to be detached whenever it is removed from its normal position in the back of the eye. And this can occur in anybody at any age. People who are experiencing retinal detachment report seeing "floaters" (dark spots that seem to move around in their field of vision) or a gray curtain moving back and forth across their eyes.

There are many reasons for detached retinas. The most familiar ones are myopia, postcataract surgeries, and traumas. Blows to the head can also create retinal detachments. In my opinion, this is another reason to avoid Lasik surgery, since it weakens the eye, creating higher chances of a retinal detachment simply by bumping your head forcefully.

If the retinal detachment is very large, you must see a physician soon, because the detachment can cause lack of blood flow to the photoreceptors and can kill them. Within a short period of time, possibly a week or two, you can lose your vision. As an exception, I met a person who received a head-butt during a violent fight in prison. As a result of the fight, his retina detached, and the prison physician was not capable of diagnosing it. Only after he had served his term was he seen by a top ophthalmologist, who told him that he had already had a detachment for several months. So he had reattachment surgery, and to his amazement, as well as his ophthalmologist's and my own, his vision returned to almost normal, and the retina was functional.

But this is extraordinary, and most of the time it doesn't happen that way. Usually, within a couple of weeks of lack of blood flow to the photoreceptors, they die. What should we do then?

A female patient came to me once, complaining of a retinal detachment in one eye and poor vision in the other. One thing I noticed was that she wasn't blinking. She told me it was written in her medical chart that she wasn't blinking, but none of her doctors had paid attention to the notation. Therefore, I told her to blink, and her vision improved very quickly after that.

Pay attention to your demeanor. Are you blinking? Are you not blinking? Do you pay attention to your retina or not?

Also, when you have a retinal detachment, make sure that you don't bend your head, or the retina can fall even more. After the healing process, it's important for you to get a lot of massage on your neck and on your back in order to bring more blood to the head and to strengthen your retina with nurturing blood flow to the eyes. But some of the exercises for loosening your neck (e.g., in the section on glaucoma) could hurt since they require you to bend your head down, which could cause damage. So in the acute time of retinal detachment, don't do movement exercises; instead, massage is the best option for you to relax the tension in your neck and back. After the detachment has healed, then it is okay to return to the movement exercises.

Some of the reasons for retinal detachment are emotional. A boy I once knew told me that, after his retinal reattachment surgery, he woke up one day and discovered he had some vision. But because his mother was not in the room, it traumatized him, and he became blind again. There are tissues that respond to our emotions, so it's very important to be as calm as you can be, even in the hardest of situations. It can preserve both your sanity and your retina!

Exercise Program for Retinal Detachment

- Look at Details (with the parts of your eyes that are *not* functioning well, by covering the parts that do see well): 10 minutes daily.
- Look into the Distance: 20 minutes daily, in 10-minute intervals.
- Palming: 24 minutes daily, 6 minutes at a time (once a week, as long as you do not have glaucoma, sit down and palm for an hour, listening to something pleasant like music or a book on tape).
- Darkness and Light Exercise: 20 minutes daily.

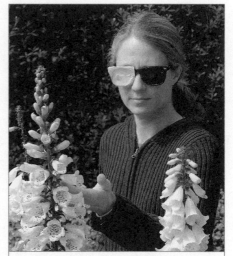

Figure 6.9. Look at details with the parts of your eyes that are *not* functioning well.

With retinal detachment, after exercising the blind or fuzzy spot, quite a few people start to have some more vision in it, which is a wonderful phenomenon. It happens because some of the cells are only dormant, even though some are dead. When we wake up the dormant cells, we have access to more vision.

Extra Exercise for Retinal Detachment: Darkness and Light

If parts of your retina are dead, or if you have a sighted eye, patch your sighted eye and with paper obstruct the parts of your disabled eye that are still functioning. Then look at the world through holes in the paper, using only the parts of your eyes that do not function well.

Four times a day, after six minutes of palming, go into a dark room. Now you will want to use blinking lights. At the School for Self-

Healing we sell small blinking lights you can use for this exercise, but any different-colored blinking lights will do. The object is simply to turn on the blinking lights to activate the parts of your eyes that are not working.

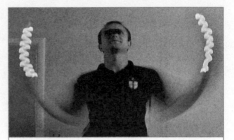

Figure 6.10. Use blinking or flashing lights in a dark room to activate the parts of the eyes that are not working.

When you have the functional parts of your eyes covered and you are looking at blinking lights in a dark room, you may not see anything at all at first. But over time you may start to see small changes in the darkness. Small flashes of light may start to occur. Be patient. In time you may start to see more and more flashing lights and, eventually, shapes may start to occur. Sometimes a picture comes; when it does, it's wonderful!

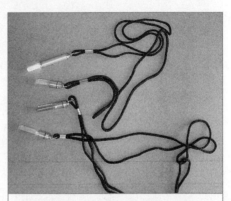

Figure 6.11. The small blinking lights we use at the school.

A much more subtle way of accomplishing this same exercise is to obstruct the functional part of your eyes and to walk outside in bright sunlight, crossing between a brightly lit area and a shaded area. Walk with somebody who can help you to make sure you do not trip. Move your

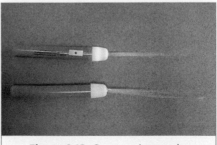

Figure 6.12. Our magic wands.

head from side to side, but do not move your eyes. The extremes of light and dark may start to become apparent over time. In this way,

155

you are accomplishing the same thing as with the blinking lights. You are activating the part of your eyes that does not function well, so that vision in your blind spot will start to develop.

If you have some vision, obstruct your strong eye with a patch and your weak eye with paper with holes cut out for the weak areas to look through. Now walk in your garden or somewhere safe, with a companion who can hold your hand or catch you if you fall, and move your head from side to side slowly so as to help you notice more details. Then take off your patches; 75 percent of people who do this will see an immediate improvement in their vision. The improvement is temporary, but repetition of this exercise makes it become stable.

Correcting Vitreous Detachment

The vitreous is the gel-like substance that covers the surface of the retina, and it is in fact attached to the retina via millions of fine, intertwined fibers. As the vitreous shrinks from age and neglect, detachment from the retina can occur.

Vitreous detachment is much more common, but less harmful, than retinal detachment. Only in rare cases does vitreous detachment lead to partial blindness. But it does lead to a tremendous amount of floaters that obstruct vision. A floater is a tiny dark spot that seems to be floating around in your field of vision, obstructing what you are looking at.

In a minority of cases, vitreous detachment can lead to retinal detachment or puckers, by pulling apart the retina; this, in turn, can lead to bleeding and flooding of the photoreceptor cells, causing blindness. But most of the time, it's relatively harmless and just leads to some floaters.

Normally, with a retinal pucker, after looking at an eye chart and seeing it to some extent, there is a sense of clarity in the rest of your visual system. If you take off the pinholes and you take off the patch, you will find that your vision is very much clearer. That's why repetition of these exercises is so useful.

If you experience vitreous detachment, however, I recommend getting checked by two or three ophthalmologists, especially retinal specialists, to be sure that the detachment didn't cause any harm to the retina at the same time.

Often, people are afraid of the floaters. A good way to deal with them might seem rather amazing and surprising. The secret is to look at them! You just walk outdoors on a very sunny day, or at least on a bright day, and look at the floaters one by one. If you cannot see them one by one because there are groups of floaters, look at them group by group. When you isolate and look at the floaters, you cause the vitreous fluid to collide against the floaters, which breaks them up and causes them to disappear.

For example, if you have more floaters in your right eye, patch or obstruct your left eye and walk for twenty minutes in the sun, somewhere with a nice view to look at. As you look at the view, floaters will appear. As they appear, look right at the floaters; as you do, the vitreous fluid will collide against them and destroy them. Normally, what happens when you look at a floater is that it floats away and then comes back; when you look at it again, your vitreous fluid hits the floater and breaks it into pieces. Then you see smaller pieces, and you look at either one of them or at several pieces, and you break them once again.

Choose a floater to look at, possibly the largest one, and when it floats away, look into the distance. Then look at that floater again when it comes back, and exercise with that floater, back and forth, every day. Most likely, after a few weeks, that floater will disappear. Then you choose the next one. Do it in a neutral state of mind; blink and breathe. If you have floaters in both eyes, but more in one eye than the other, patch the eye with fewer floaters and look at the floaters with the other eye.

I had a patient named Tony who had laser surgeries, retinal detachment, and terrible vitreous floaters. Moreover, he couldn't drive. His doctor had mistakenly told him to wear sunglasses. That only made the floaters worse. I told him to do a lot of sunning, to walk, and to look at the floaters. I will never forget the time I walked with him up and down a hill around my previous office. He looked at plants, he looked at the view, and very quickly he improved his vision from 20/200 with glasses to 20/20 with glasses; he also reduced his diopter level significantly, from 13 to 8 diopters.

Tony reduced his myopia and reduced the floaters, and his vision is perfect now compared to how it used to be; it is better without his glasses, and it's better with his glasses, and with much less correction. (This wonderful man volunteered to have his picture taken as the model on my DVD, *Yoga for Your Eyes*, which has helped many people to see better.)

Tony used the internal forces of his own body to improve his eyes, and the improvement was massive. You can do the same. Your internal forces are only partially known, and they're stronger than what anyone can imagine.

Even though many floaters are not a result of vitreous detachment, the treatment is the same. You have to mentally accept the fact that it's okay for you to have this floater; then you have to look at it. If you've lived with floaters for many years and it's familiar to you, it will probably be hard for your mind to believe they can disappear. If it is one floater, look at it. If there are groups of floaters, look only at one group. If it is a big floater, look at one part of it. Repeated exercises will show you that you can actually decrease it, change its shape and, with time, rid yourself of it. The only thing that keeps the floater going is your disgust for that floater and lack of willingness to look at it. That's what happens with most people. We have forces within us that can destroy that which impedes us, if we only let them do it.

Additionally, what we learn from the fact that we are experiencing vitreous detachment in the first place is that the health of the eye is going in the wrong direction. Therefore, once we eliminate the floaters, we must return to the basic eye exercises in the beginning of this book in order to strengthen and heal the entire eye.

Correcting Macular Puckers and Holes

Some people suddenly discover they can no longer see centrally. It's a scary situation. From such a person's viewpoint, one day he or she sees perfectly, and the next day his or her central vision has disappeared. When the person meets an ophthalmologist, the ophthalmologist has absolutely nothing to offer except sympathy.

Often, this situation is caused by macular holes and macular puckers—basically, detachment of the vitreous that takes with it a part of the macula. Other times, we simply have cells that have withered and died. In all cases, the treatment is the same.

Exercise Program for Macular Puckers and Holes: 80 Minutes a Day

- Palming: 24 minutes daily, 6 minutes at a time.
- Sunning: 30 minutes daily, in three 10-minute intervals.
- Skying (if there is no sun): 8 minutes daily.
- Long Swing: 5 minutes daily.
- Pinhole Glasses: 10 minutes daily.

Remember not to simply take one part of the day and do your eye exercises all at once. The best results come from working on your eyes all the time, throughout your day. Find a few minutes

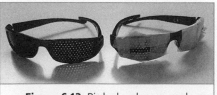

Figure 6.13. Pinhole glasses and pinhole glasses with obstruction.

here and there and let the eye exercises in this book find their way naturally into your routine. Thus, vision improvement will become part of your daily life in an organic way. This is the way to improve for the long term.

Extra Exercise for Macular Puckers and Holes: Pinhole Glasses

Put the pinhole glasses on and then cover the eye that sees normally. Use the eye that has the macular hole in it to look straight ahead at an eye chart. You should put the eye chart in full light, preferably sunlight. The pinhole glasses will protect you from the temporary glare, and your tendency will be to tilt your head to see. Don't tilt your head; instead, look straight ahead. Then close your eyes and remember exactly how the letters looked to you.

At times, you will see only the very big letter from a very short distance. If that's what you see, it's okay. Allow that area of your eye to be functional. After you remember the exact shape and contour of the letter or letters that you saw, open your eyes and look again.

Now move your head very slightly from side to side, no more than half a centimeter. That's enough for you to see the letter moving in the opposite direction from the way *you* are moving, through the fuzz or the veil that you are looking through.

The next step is to put masking tape on the pinhole lens covering the area that would be the central periphery, and do the same exercise.

Normally, when you have a macular pucker, you see better peripherally. So next, cover the entire lens over the weaker eye

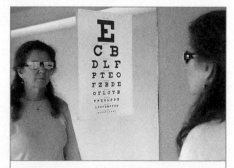

Figure 6.14. Use the eye that has the macular hole in it to look straight ahead at an eye chart.

with construction paper that has only a tiny hole, made by a pen or pencil, right where the main blind spot is in your vision. Now look at the eye chart through that pinhole you made.

Note: It is dangerous to create a hole in the paper while you are wearing these glasses. Do not create the hole while the paper is on your face. Even though it seems easiest to do it this way (since only then can you test whether the hole is in the correct spot), it is best to find the blind spot and to create the hole on the paper when it is away from your eyes. It may take you a few tries until the hole is positioned right in front of the fuzzy or blind spot, but do not do it in front of your face, even if it seems more convenient to do so.

Sometimes it's impossible to see any print through the hole. If that is the case with your vision, you should start this exercise by stimulating that area with blinking lights like the ones you can order through our School for Self-Healing in San Francisco.

With a macular pucker, some cells are still alive, but they are dormant in most cases, and they're not being activated. Looking at the eye chart with only the fuzzy area in your central field will clarify your vision. Even slight clarification can make a big difference to your visual system because it eases the burden on the rest of the cells.

Correcting Retinitis Pigmentosa

Note: If you have turned to this section because you have retinitis pigmentosa, you should not read on without a broader understanding of our approach. Please go back to the beginning of the book and work from there onward. Be aware of all the deep concepts of life, vitality, and vision. Then you will be ready to work with this section.

Retinitis pigmentosa is an inherited disease characterized by a gradual, progressive degeneration of the retina. This leads to loss of peripheral vision and night vision difficulties and can also lead to central vision loss as well.

If you know that you are predisposed to retinitis pigmentosa, you should start to work on shifting and peripheral vision exercises at a very young age. If you did this, you would simply be diagnosed as having some missing spots in your visual system, but you would basically see well.

Although retinitis pigmentosa is genetic in nature, it is exacerbated by the normal stresses in life. What are our stresses? It is stressful when you look at someone and can see only their head and not the rest of them. It is even more stressful to see everything fuzzy. Another major source of stress is caused by the vision loss itself. It is especially stressful when you see well enough to get by, but not well enough to function fully. You may walk on the street and see people, but you don't recognize your friend's face immediately. Mental stress occurs from people having their feelings hurt by that, and from you criticizing yourself about it, even though you would forgive anyone else for not being able to see someone's face.

I think it's very important to announce to the world, "I do have an eye disease, and if you want me to recognize you, just say, 'Here I am.' Sometimes don't say it; see first if I recognize you and then, only if I don't, say, 'Here I am.' And if I do recognize you, that's a great thing. I'm seeing you, and you acknowledged that."

Let people know that there is suffering involved in your life, and don't have them feel bad or guilty about it. You'd be amazed how much people's intelligence grows when they understand how to treat other people—and how much it shrinks when you hide a phenomenon that you are experiencing.

From the very first year that I had started to work on overcoming my blindness while also working on others, I found out that those people who hide a serious problem always suffer for it. Even if they have a good reason to hide (i.e., because they would be fired from work), at the end of the day, they still suffer more from hiding than from revealing it.

Other people revere their problems and use them as a crutch or as a tool to gain favors; they try to get others to do special things for them that they wouldn't have done had they not known of a problem. Those people don't heal either.

The people who heal are the ones who look at the problem as a matter of fact. I could be short, I could be tall, I could have cataracts, I could have retinitis pigmentosa, I could limp; either way, I'm a whole person, I'm okay, and I just have to deal with my problems as well as my triumphs. The problem becomes much less of a problem when it's being discussed.

Exercise Program for Retinitis Pigmentosa

- Palming: 24 minutes daily.
- Sunning: 20 minutes daily.
- Night Walking: 1 hour, twice a week (if possible).
- Shifting: 10 minutes daily.
- Extra Exercises: 20 minutes daily.

Sometimes night walking is not possible because your vision is not strong enough in the dark. In this case you cannot walk at night. The ability to night walk could come as a result of improvement in your peripheral vision.

There's a big difference between simply sitting in a dark room and actually walking around in the dark. The body is meant to respond to visual information; therefore the brain receives the impulses much better through movement in the dark than through being still.

If your vision isn't clear enough at night—and so many people with retinitis pigmentosa lose that capacity—you may still see well enough to adapt to your room with some light from the outside. In that case, spend about an hour each night for the next six months exercising in the following sequence: first walk back and forth in your room; then sit cross-legged on the floor (occasionally moving in a rotating motion just enough to create the sensation of movement); finally, walk forward and backward again. This should begin to stimulate some cells that are just dormant and not dead. If you do that, there's a good chance you will slow down the retinitis pigmentosa greatly, and eventually develop good enough night vision to go night walking.

I will never forget a man in his forties who came to me with retinitis pigmentosa. His mother had lost her vision to retinitis pigmentosa, the same way he did. His vision was very clear when he looked at an eye chart: it was 20/30 with his glasses on, which was within the normal range; peripherally, he didn't even have 3 percent vision. Whenever he would enter a slightly darker room, he would be blind momentarily. So I taught him to palm for fifteen seconds whenever he stepped into a dark room. When he took his hands from his eyes, he saw much better.

In order to improve his peripheral vision, we created an exercise that required three assistants but ended up being very successful. Remember that the periphery senses movement and the central vision mainly senses a still picture. The exercise we created made use of this principle in a dynamic way. I had one assistant stand in front of the patient and throw a ball back and forth to him. While they played catch, I had two more assistants stand on either side of the man, throwing a ball back and forth across his field of vision. So these tennis balls were crossing each other in the backyard. Slowly, he started to notice the ball going side to side more and more. It was gradual, but he was becoming more aware of the periphery.

After four days of intensive training, his peripheral vision improved to 85 percent. Now, there's no question that even though the treatment was very intensive and fruitful, the therapy did not regenerate 80 to 82 percent of his peripheral field in four days. In all likelihood, what had happened was that though many cells had already died, most others were simply dormant, and by doing the work that we did, we woke up the dormant cells, thus helping him to regain and to maintain his vision for many years. Later that year, he reported to us that he no longer bumped his head against airplane compartments and that he was able to see when students in his classes raised their hands. He had been superintendent of education for Michigan, and whenever he visited classes before, when he looked straight ahead, he wouldn't see anyone who had been raising a hand. Now he could.

So whenever you move to a differently lit room, palm. Put your hands over your eye orbits and visualize that you're seeing darkness, or maybe even blackness. Breathe deeply and slowly. The breathing will bring you oxygen and relaxation. The palming will widen your pupils and will allow the healthy cells in your retina to function better.

Extra Exercises for Retinitis Pigmentosa

The Mask of Zorro

A minority of people with retinitis pigmentosa see better peripherally and worse centrally. Other people lose their vision almost completely. In each case, it's very important for us to work on ourselves, confronting our own personal manifestation of the problem, patiently and frequently.

If you lost most of your central vision to retinitis pigmentosa, place construction paper with a hole poked out in the area of your central vision over your eye. Walk in daylight, whether in the garden or in the street, with someone who will hold your hand, unless you're independent enough. Even though you blocked the vision that you use most of the time, observe all the details that you can see. Look at smaller details than the ones you can easily see. So, on the one hand, you would say, "I already have a much smaller portion of the picture." But, at the same time, you want to build a sense of central vision. Central vision is such that we always look at smaller details than the ones we see.

Look at smaller and smaller and smaller details, and you will start to see them better and better. Walk with the paper on your eye for a minimum of forty minutes a day, and a maximum of a hundred minutes a day. At first, you may not be able to tolerate the paper for more than ten minutes at a time; do it just eight minutes at a time, and never strain. Always palm before you do it; sometimes palm in the middle of doing it; and often palm after you finish your walk. Look straight ahead while you walk.

Some people laughingly call this exercise "The Mask of Zorro." So, walk with the Mask of Zorro and observe all the details you can see through it. You're giving yourself a chance to wake up all the dormant cells in the center of your retina.

One thing you need to remember is that memory is a powerful tool. Whatever you look at, as fuzzy as it may appear (due to the cells that were destroyed), if you close your eyes and remember it exactly how you saw it, when you open your eyes, it will be at least a tad clearer, and sometimes much more so.

After a few weeks of closing your eyes and remembering what you saw, close your eyes and remember contrast. So, if you look at white flowers versus green leaves, close your eyes and say, "The flowers are white, the leaves are green" and, in your mind, visualize the flowers to be an even brighter white and the leaves to be an even darker green. In addition, you could visualize greater sharpness of the different colors that you saw. You could look at the sky and say, "The sky is bright blue, and the clouds are white." To create as much contrast as you could, close your eyes and say, "The ocean is blue, and the waves are white." The imagery has to come with a sense of realistic colors.

Then visualize larger objects. Visualize that the petals of a flower are large and distinct, even though they may look small or almost nonexistent with the poor vision you have. Visualize a greater amount of details than the amount of details that you saw with your eyes open.

When you look with the area that is nearly blind, the most important thing is to look through it as if that's all you can see with. Many people are very disturbed with the whole concept of looking with an area that is damaged. But that's where healing begins: where you accept exactly the space that you are in. Nurturing your weakest area and feeling okay with it will strengthen every part of your life. You will take away the pressure on the rest of your visual system, and it will be easier for you to use your eyes. Parts of your brain that are no longer active, because of lack of stimuli from the exact blind spots, will start to work.

You will gain back some of the normal vision in the blind spot. Sometimes the blind spot decreases, and you can slowly control and manage your vision. The loss you would have experienced over a period of five years stretches to a period of twenty-five years, and your visual life becomes more normal and more predictable.

Waving Lights in the Dark

If walking outside in the starlight or moonlight is way too difficult and above your capacity, and your central vision is good or even excellent, then sit in a dark room and turn lights on and off. At the School for Self-Healing we use fiber-optic lights, which look like many strands of plastic spaghetti sticking out from the end of a plastic wand. The wand projects a light that causes the strands to light up in many different colors. They turn on and off, and we can wave them sideways. The good thing about fiber-optic lights is that when you wave them—we call them magic wands—it stimulates your peripheral vision, provided you're looking forward. In the past we would put down newspapers to protect the floor from falling wax because we used candles for this exercise.

If you wave either a fiber-optic light or a candle in the dark, the movement will wake up many of the dormant cells you have. The benefit of the flame from a candle is that it moves, and the movement of the flame activates the rods of the retina. What's good about fiber-optic lights is that you can wave them. Also, they have stronger light than candles and do not drip wax. Sometimes, however, the fiber-optic lights are too strong for the eyes to exercise and improve as compared to candles.

Spending positive time with your eyes will eliminate the negativity you hear about or experience with them. I once had a patient who came to me in San Francisco from Australia. She was able to improve her central vision from nearsightedness to nearly normal vision and did not need glasses to look straight ahead, but she had severe retinitis pigmentosa. For ten years she did not walk freely outdoors at night, but she did walk freely outdoors in the daytime. After she practiced waving lights in the dark, and also having extensive amounts of massage, she was able to walk at night on dark streets for the first time.

After a few weeks of this exercise, gradually start to use small, medium, and large pieces of paper taped to the bridge of your nose. Wave the fiber-optic lights to the sides of your eyes, and you may get a sense that one eye sees more light than the other eye. If this is the case, close the eye that sees more light for a short while (about five or six seconds), and use only the other eye; then open both eyes and use both. The idea is to create evenness between the two eyes and to make the brain immediately use peripheral vision.

Sometimes, the fiber-optic lights will not be visible. Other times, people with retinitis pigmentosa will not notice the color of the lights. So it is better to start with red blinking lights because red has the longest light waves, making it the easiest light to see. Then, over time, you can change to different colors.

Truly, anytime someone is experiencing a blind spot, blinking lights and fiber-optic lights in a dark room can bring to life the parts of the eye that are not functioning. In this way, you start to create that process of slowly expanding that which you are capable of doing.

A Final Note about Peripheral Exercises

If you have retinitis pigmentosa, no matter what condition your eyes are in, make it a habit to notice the periphery throughout the day. Work the periphery every waking moment. Wave your hands in your periphery for a few seconds at a time throughout the day. This way, the two eyes will be working together. In the center, one eye can dominate; with the periphery, however, both eyes must work, so one eye cannot dominate the other.

When you wave your hands to the sides of your eyes and close one eye, you see only one hand waving. Close the other eye, and you see only the other hand waving. Open both eyes, and you see both hands waving. This way you know that both eyes are working together.

Chapter 7

The Blind Spots of Conventional Wisdom

The Hidden Danger of Sunglasses

It has become common for people in our culture to put on sunglasses as soon as they step out of the house on a sunny day. People see the sun as some sort of enemy that is about to cause harm to their eyes. Doctors warn us of the dangers of sun exposure, and there certainly are reasons to take the proper precautions to protect our bodies from too much exposure to ultraviolet light. Our eyes, however, are made to function at their highest and best when they are exposed to a full range of light and darkness.

It's important to be in touch with our bodies on a cellular level. You can't normally see your cells unless you have microscopic pictures taken of them and are able to look at the pictures. We tend to ignore our body and our body parts. But it is very important to have a very thorough feel for our own body.

Enjoy the sun and also the dark of night. Seldom wear sunglasses because they weaken the pupils. Enjoy the sun throughout the day, and don't use a flashlight when you take a walk at night. Enjoy the expansion of the pupils at night. Make your eyes more vital and more alive. Give your eyes a sense of love so that, in many ways, you love your life and you love the universe. Allow your eyes to develop good fixation, which is the ability to allow the proper amount of light to enter the pupils in order to see better in whatever situation you find yourself. When your pupils become firmer and not sluggish, you can then have a better fixation and allow the exact amount of light you need for your sight to improve.

In the daytime, you will end up seeing details seeing details *with* much greater clarity. This will take the load and distress away from other parts of the visual system, like the retina and the lens. At night-time, your pupils will be wide enough to see all that is around you in the dark. Your whole system will become stronger as a result of your pupils being able to absorb more light.

Ignoring your eyes, and not giving them enough darkness or enough light, will weaken the system through the years. Renewing our strength by reducing the amount of time we wear sunglasses, and reducing the amount of time we spend indoors, can make a huge difference.

Be wary of the sun scare.

Many people do not realize that there are pigments in the eyes that darken the light. *Melanin pigment* is in the choroid area, the area that nourishes the retina. One of the ten layers of the retina is melanin. So the retina itself has a whole layer of melanin pigment that darkens the light. Therefore, you have "sunglasses" inside the retina itself! When you wear sunglasses, it takes away the usefulness of this layer in the retina. It also darkens the light as it arrives at the retina, so you do not use your own pigments to darken the light. Consequently, your pigments migrate to the back of the retina and are not as effective as they could have been otherwise.

Believe it or not, sunglasses hurt your retina just as much as crutches can hurt one's legs. If your legs are weak and you are too quick to use a cane or crutches or braces to walk with, you may never give up your crutches. But if you work very hard on strengthening your legs, there is a possibility you will regain their full use. In some cases there isn't such a possibility, and that's when crutches or braces are very useful. But if it's at all possible for you to strengthen your legs yourself, do not use crutches as a method of healing, since it's best to work on the body's independence.

The same is true for sunglasses. The more you use sunglasses, the weaker your pupils become. You are also weakening the defense mechanism that exists in your retina and that has existed in your ancestors' retinas for millions of years.

If, on the other hand, you practice sunning for at least twenty minutes a day, you will find that your eyes adjust much better to the sun. The sun, throughout the years, will become very comfortable for you. You will also find that darkness is easier for you to handle. As your pupils grow wider and your retinal cells become more sensitive, the dark will not appear to be as dark. Best of all, you will enjoy opening your eyes wide in both the strongest and the weakest lights. You will also be happier because the combination of the sun's rays and the hemoglobin in the blood releases many hormones and neural transmitters, such as serotonin, that lead to a sense of joy. You will probably also have an easier time releasing melatonin at night without taking any vitamins or drugs, simply because of your good sun exposure. The joy of this will lead to many other good things in your life.

If your eyes are sun-sensitive and do not widen enough in the dark, the other mechanisms, even if they're healthy, may not function to the best of their potential. Most of what the visual system does consists of absorbing light and processing it. Therefore, it's important that that process be easy and relaxing for the body.

The Dangers of Corrective Lenses

There are three essential dangers from utilizing corrective lenses. If you wear glasses, you tend not to use as much of your external muscles because you depend on a focal point. For this reason, you weaken them throughout the years, which is very bad for your total mechanism.

If you wear contact lenses, your body wants to reject them at first because they are foreign objects. This means you must weaken the immune system in your eyes in order to accept the contacts. This weakens the entire eye over time. Also, the contacts prevent enough oxygen from coming to the eyes, because the contact lenses block it. Even permeable contact lenses are not permeable enough for oxygen.

And whether you wear glasses or contacts, the biggest danger is simply the sense of dependency you create. The more you wear them, the more you need them. You never give your eyes the chance to work out and to regain their sense of strength and natural ability.

At the age of forty-five, seven out of eight people wear corrective lenses. I don't think we were born to have all this correction. The reason that we have all this correction is that we are creatures of imitation.

There are many millions of brain cells that work only to imitate each other. Monkeys imitate each other, and humans imitate other humans. By practicing vision improvement and being adamant about it, you will be able to affect your vision and the world for the better. This book will change the world completely because many boundaries will break in what we believe our real capacity is. Just imagine how many diseases will be prevented as a result of people working on their eyes.

Now you know how to improve your own vision. You have an eye chart on the wall. Let's assume that you read the fourth line with great ease, and then you read the fifth, sixth, and seventh with more difficulty. By the eighth, you can't read anymore. If this is true, you're standing exactly in the right place. It could be three, five, ten, or twenty feet. As your vision improves, you'll be able to stand farther away.

Now also determine five or six different objects in your environment that you like to look at. These objects could be flowers from three yards away, or a fence from a yard or two. Changeable items like the clouds in the sky cannot measure your improvement, but steady objects, with steady light at the same time of the day, can. As you improve your vision, you will be able to see more details in these objects.

When you reduce your prescription and first see with a weaker prescription, just be aware of the fact that you will not see as well initially. Normally, you will improve within three weeks. Keep the glasses in your pocket all the time, but try to see well without them as long as it feels effortless. Don't squint or strain. Just look softly through the fog or fuzziness you have and work on your mind to reduce your frustration.

The most important thing to remember is that how we train ourselves to look is more important, for the time being, than what we see. With time, what we see will be more important. You're returning to the process of looking. When you were an infant, you didn't see things well, and you didn't care, because you did not know that things could be seen any better than how you saw them. As you looked at details, from one to the other, your vision got better. Your macula, the fovea centralis inside it, and even the foveola (which is a smaller spot within the fovea that sees details), started to act well because your mind was interested in what you were looking at. As a result, the connection between the brain and eye became stronger. Slowly, as you started to crawl and walk, the brain developed, and the eyes became stronger, seeing better and better. Normally, childhood vision is much better than adult vision. Many people measure childhood vision as 20/15, which is better than 20/20.

We want to return to that phase. We want to look with great curiosity at all the details the world gives us. Some are nice, and some are ugly, but we always want to look.

A woman who started to lose her vision stated in one of my classes, "I stopped having any interest in looking at things because, in my opinion, the city I live in is ugly." I could understand why she stopped looking at details, but the more we look consciously at details, the better we see them. There are many people who live in a beautiful city like San Francisco, and still do not look at details. Remember: all details, whether beautiful or not, could be interesting. Remember that when you were an infant, all details were interesting to you.

Looking through your fog could be interesting as well. For example, you can look at the different details in flowers from a distance where you can see the flowers relatively well; then look away, either at a fence, a bush, the sky, or buildings that are farther away, but on which you still see some details. Close your eyes and visualize the contrast between details at a far distance. You can visualize the leaf of a bush and the sky, the fence and the earth, or whatever could have different contrasts. Then look at the objects again, and return to the flowers. Many people will see the flowers better.

Straining your eyes to look far makes you see worse; looking far without strain, with the help of your imagination, and with the help of seeing more and more details, allows you to see better nearby. Nearsighted people need to work on slowly making the point of focus farther away. This means that a nearsighted person who sees really well from 20 centimeters should hope that, after beginning this practice, he or she will see really well from 25 and then 30 centimeters. It is the ability to see farther and farther at a distance, even if it is from a relatively close range, that is going to heal your myopia.

So, the number one thing to remember is, when you put your glasses in your pocket, don't worry about identifying people's faces. Announce to all your friends, relatives, and family that you have decided to spend the next four to six months using your glasses as little as possible in order to improve your vision problems. The main thing is to make sure that when you look at the world, you look at it from the eyes with which you were born. Make sure that you blink. Adjust to the world as it is. Enjoy it.

Keep in mind that if your tendency is to wear glasses, you can improve your vision enough that glasses won't be necessary. In fact, you may end up seeing better *without* them than you had originally been seeing *with* them. If you have recovered from a major eye surgery with rehabilitation, instead of just seeing the top of the chart with your glasses, you may see the bottom of the chart with your glasses. If you cannot recover your vision, you may learn how to use the little vision that you have to function as fully as you can with your eyes and body. There is a possibility for rehabilitation in every situation, and we need to believe in our eyes to create such a revolution. This revolution will come from the simple truth that we have inner powers and that this book has helped you to reach them. With diligence, faith, love, and work, we will be able to change ourselves and all who are around us, until this world is a better place.

The Real Cost of Vision Problems

As I have pointed out, the medical establishment has few answers for most of our common eye disorders. Even so, it is important to ask: even if reliable and safe treatments did exist, who would pay for them?

It is my opinion that the time has come for all of us to ask what the real cost of vision problems is—not just in terms of money, but also in terms of productivity, quality of life, and morale. When someone loses his eyesight, his entire life is affected, along with the lives of everyone he knows. It isn't just one person's problem; it is society's problem. The reality is that by neglecting each other, we neglect ourselves; and, in the end, we all pay dearly.

I hope we all realize that the trend in developed and developing nations is not toward bigger budgets for vision care. On the contrary, very little money is currently spent by cities, states, and nations on the vision care of their citizenry, and even less will likely be spent in the future.

Sadly, there is no help coming from the medical profession to reinforce strength in the eyes. And most people harbor the false belief that their eyes cannot get better. Therefore, we need to start with new seeds of hope until most people in the world are willing to work on their eyes. In fact, we need a silent but continuous revolution. This goes beyond countries or flags. To believe in ourselves and in our eyes is to open a window to our heart. With continuous work on the eyes, we can make a huge difference in our self-image and in resolving many other problems—personal, national, and international.

The positive reinforcement comes with positive results. Think about it. We relinquished our power to acute care, which is a false promise for the health of our eyes. When you do so for one problem, the next one often appears rather quickly. The truth is that if we ourselves took good care of our eyes, the few times that we would need acute care, it would work just fine, and we would also rehabilitate quicker.

Because physicians think that nothing can be fixed in the eye except by the mechanical acute care of which they're capable, they are not researching the vital forces of the eyes. But we have several vital forces. We have the macula, which will start to be more active when linked with the mind. We have our minds, which can reinforce much better vision through imagery and memory. We have our lenses, which become much more flexible when we balance their use. We have our pupils, which become stronger if they contract much in the sun or daylight and expand much at nighttime. We can also have good circulation, with which we could improve and refresh the eyes and prevent most aging problems related to vision.

The truth of the matter is that it's very important to create great internal changes. Sometimes this requires that you change or widen your whole being. You can acquire new skills that you didn't have before, ones that are exciting and useful to you. These may be skills of any kind. There are more than 87,000 professions on earth. Even if you don't change your profession, you could learn new ways of operating and functioning. If you change your profession, do it with grace and ease. Another important thing is that many people are already at the end of their careers. They have accomplished their goals at work by the age of forty-five or fifty. It is wonderful to see, especially in the United States, so many people in their forties, fifties, and sixties returning to school to acquire new knowledge and skills.

It is important on an emotional level that you have something to look forward to in life, that you feel your life is meaningful, and that every moment of your life is creative. This emotional advancement is the background of healing. It's hard to heal if you resent your own life. It is easier to heal if you feel that you have something to look forward to. This way you can help the world and yourself at the same time. It motivates you to invest in the time that it takes to improve your vision. It gives you the vigilance to maintain your improvement as time goes on. It gives you the impetus to feel well enough within yourself to change for the better.

Your happiness is precious. It comes with self-acceptance, and there is no better time than in your forties, fifties, and sixties to work on self-acceptance. When we have self-acceptance, we place less importance on adding extra weight or on the wrinkles that come with age. This is a time when we like all we've done, all we are currently doing, and all we will be doing. Believe me, our beauty will reflect itself. A straight face with no wrinkles does not match a wrinkled face with great happiness. A thin and fit Hollywood body is not nearly as attractive as an energetic body, even if the latter appears to be imperfect. At this particular time in life, working on a sense of inner happiness and working on a particular part of our body are parallel goals. Working on our flexibility and devoting ourselves to expanding our thoughts are comparable to each other. Slowly but surely, your vision will get better and better. If you keep shifting and looking at details, you will maintain the vigilance of thought and the emotional openness required. This kind of maturity is our next step in life.

So, what we need is to inform ourselves, to work with ourselves, to convince others, to suggest support groups, and to suggest change in the world, bringing it to the consciousness of everyone we meet. Explain to them that it's time for us to be aware of our powers. Who knows, maybe as a result of what you do, new research will spring up in your hometown, and it will make this a much better world than the one we live in. Unlike what most people believe, our world is not as developed as it could be. Our eyes, which are so precious to us, could see so much better along with those of every human being on earth.

I'm the one to tell you that. I could have been blind right now, but I can read this book. And why? Simply because I worked on myself.

This is why it is more important than ever to spread the word that it is possible for us to take care of our own vision. It can be done in such a way that we never develop devastating eye problems in the first place, so that we never have to rely on the inadequate and antiquated approaches of our governments or of the corporate medical establishment.

The way to solve the crisis of low-or-no-budget vision care is to heal our eyes ourselves. Learn the basic exercises in *Vision for Life*. Become aware of the erosive habits you may be developing from staring at a computer screen all day and a television screen all night. Learn to blink. Learn to breathe correctly. Learn to relax. Learn to give massages so you and your loved ones can help each other maintain good blood flow along with a relaxed, confident, and radiant state of being.

This is the path to a sustainable future for our eyes. This is my vision for life.

Index

Acknowledgments

I began this book by speaking into a cassette recorder, and what I said was transcribed word for word onto paper. To translate from the spoken word into written material is not easy and, in fact, my dictation was not something one could easily convey in words, something pictorial and easily described; it was more like lyrical prose, and needed a lot of work in order to become a comprehensive tool for the reader. Yet, when I considered all the wonderful people my method had enabled me to help and the exciting new discoveries they had experienced, and when I thought about the hope I wanted to give to billions of people in the world along with my own patients, with the help of many, I began the real work of putting a book together.

Therefore, I thank Phillip Barcio for helping to compile the materials and making my ideas more comprehensible. Next, I would very much like to thank my friend Richard Mandrachio, whose talents as an editor helped enormously in presenting the book in a straightforward manner that all readers can understand and practice with. I also wish to give many thanks to photographer Richard Miller, who himself benefited tremendously from this work; he improved his vision in spite of a birth defect and a condition that caused a major loss of his optic nerve. He regained much of his vision and, through black and white pictures, was able to bring to life many of the exercises that will help you, the reader. The person to whom I extend my heartfelt gratitude more than anyone else is my good friend Jan Albin, who worked tirelessly for countless hours on all the forms the manuscript has taken. Jan offered an incredible amount of aid in editing this book and was instrumental in getting it published. Finally, my sincere thanks go to the editors and good people at North Atlantic Books who accepted my manuscript for publication.

About the Author

M EIR SCHNEIDER had the unusual misfortune to be born with cataracts and many other conditions that affected his vision; after five unsuccessful surgeries, he expected to be blind for life. Though he read only Braille, at age seventeen he began a regimen of eye exercises and healed himself of congenital blindness. Today he holds an unrestricted California driver's license.

Schneider went on to help many people improve their vision from situations that had previously been considered hopeless. He affirms his viewpoint that nearsightedness, farsightedness, astigmatism, and computer-use problems can all be prevented or overcome through his method. Schneider's innovative work in the holistic health field, especially concerning the empowerment of the individual, is an inspiring message as well as a practical guide. Many of Schneider's past students are currently practicing his method in Brazil and have become well known for their impressive work, frequently appearing on television and in popular lectures. Moreover, conventional specialists have praised Schneider's method because they saw results that exceeded their expectations. And no resistance or opposition of any kind has ever stopped Schneider from bringing his work to more and more people.

In his quest for self-improvement, Schneider discovered that the same principles by which he gained functional vision could also be applied to the entire body. This became the basis for the Meir Schneider Method of Self-Healing through Bodywork and Movement—a nonmedical, holistic health rehabilitation and prevention system. It teaches us how to use muscles and joints in a balanced way, thus preventing common degenerative conditions that arise from lifestyle, employment, injury, and health problems. This is achieved by isolating muscle groups, relaxing chronically overused muscles, stimulating brain-body neural connections, and, most importantly, enhancing circulation.

A globally respected pioneer, therapist, and educator, Meir Schneider is also the best-selling author of *The Natural Vision Improvement Kit, Yoga for the Eyes, Meir Schneider's Miracle Eyesight Method, A Lesson for Life* (also known as *Self-Healing: My Life and Vision*), *Movement for Self-Healing,* and *The Handbook for Self-Healing.* Schneider was also awarded a PhD in the Healing Arts for his work with muscular dystrophy.

In 1980 Schneider founded the School for Self-Healing, a nonprofit center in San Francisco, California, that offers educational programs through which people can improve their vision as well as other physical handicaps. Meanwhile, Schneider has trained thousands worldwide, receiving international attention for his work in the healing arts. During more than 120,000 clinical hours over the last forty-two years, he has helped people to prevent blindness and conditions like glaucoma and cataracts. Through lectures, Schneider has taught many people the principles described in detail in this book: how to activate the powerful forces of nature within the body and how to improve vision by connecting to those forces through light, movement, and relaxation. This same connection encompasses the circulation, the nervous system, the visual apparatus, and the link between the eyes and the brain.